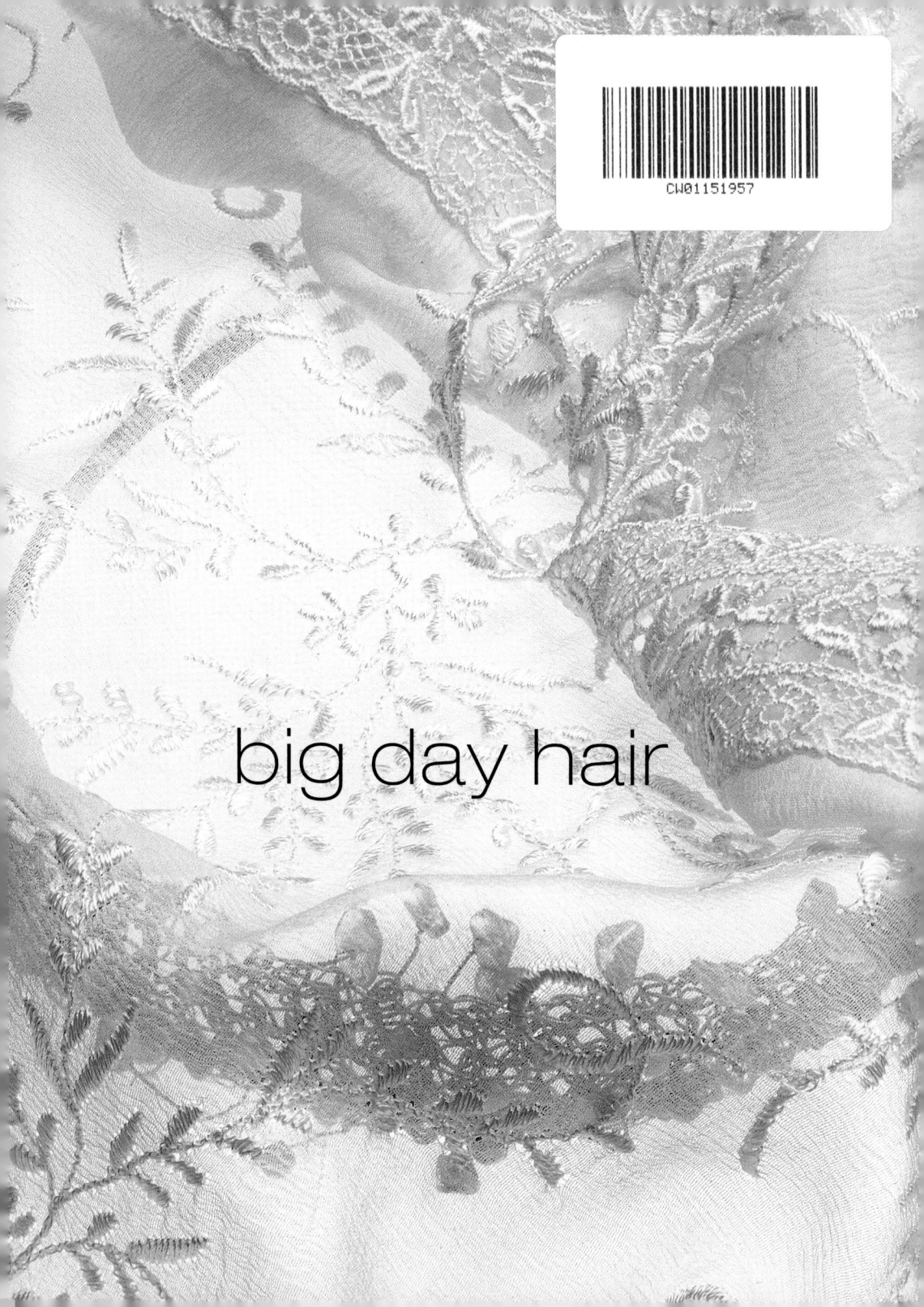

big day hair

THIS IS A CARLTON BOOK

Design, text and photography copyright © 2001 Carlton Books Limited
Original idea and concept copyright © 2001 Charles Worthington Limited

This edition published by Carlton Books Limited 2001
20 Mortimer Street
London W1T 3JW

This book is sold subject to the condition that it shall not, by way of trade or otherwise, be lent, resold, hired out or otherwise circulated without the publisher's prior written consent in any form of cover or binding other than that in which it is published and without a similar condition including this condition being imposed upon the subsequent purchaser.

All rights reserved

A CIP catalogue record for this book is available from the British Library

ISBN paperback 1 84222 200 7
ISBN hardback 1 84222 258 9

The author, licensor and publisher have made every effort to ensure that all information is correct and up to date at the time of publication. Neither the author, licensor or publisher can accept responsibility for any accident, injury or damage that results from using the ideas, information or advice offered.

The application and quality of hair products and treatments, herbal preparations and essential oils is beyond the control of the above parties, who cannot be held responsible for any problems resulting from their use. Always follow the manufacturer's instructions and, if in doubt, seek further advice.

Do not use herbal preparations or essential oils without prior consultation with a qualified practitioner or medical doctor if you are pregnant, taking any form of medication, or if you suffer from oversensitive skin. Half-doses of essential oils should always be used for children and the elderly.

No resemblance is intended to any person, living or dead, in the fiction element of this book. The events and the characters who take part in them have no relation to actual events or living people.

Writer: Lisa Helmanis
Photographer (model): Hugh Arnold
Photographer (still life): Patrice de Villiers
Illustrator: Jason Brooks
Stylist: Rachel Davis
Make-up: Chase Aston
Editorial Manager: Venetia Penfold
Art Director: Penny Stock
Senior Art Editor: Barbara Zuñiga
Commissioning Editor: Zia Mattocks
Production Controller: Janette Davis

Printed and bound in Italy

# big day hair

Charles Worthington

CARLTON
BOOKS

# contents

foreword  5

1 choose your style  8

2 get the look  26

3 the big day  64

acknowledgements  80

# foreword

Your wedding day is the most important day of your life, so then more than at any other time, you'll want your hair to be looking as stunning as the rest of you. Whatever type of wedding you're having – an ultra-modern urban do in a converted warehouse, a relaxed beach wedding in Bali or a traditional church affair – you should think of your hair as your greatest accessory. *Big Day Hair* caters for your every hair need to make sure you have perfect hair for your perfect day. As well as advice on how to identify the hairstyle that best suits your face shape, dress and accessories, it offers advice on how to get your hair in peak condition in the run up to the big day. It is also packed with great hairstyles – everything from the most chic, sleek updo to the most romantic tumbling tresses – for every type of wedding, from boho vintage, classic and country to fashionista, beach and rock chic. There are also lots of essential tips for making your style last through the day, as well as ideas for easy transformations for the reception and going away.

*Charles Worthington*

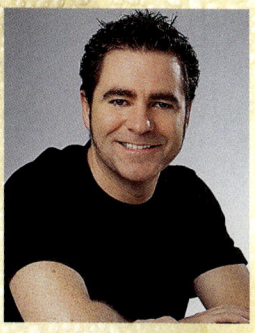
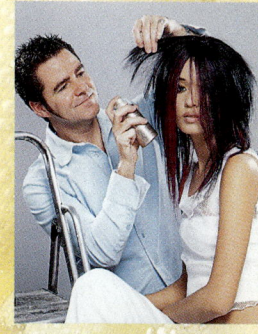
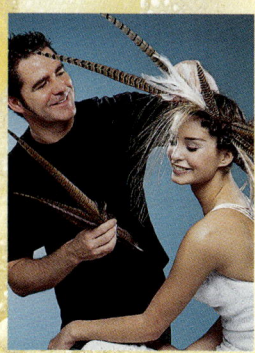

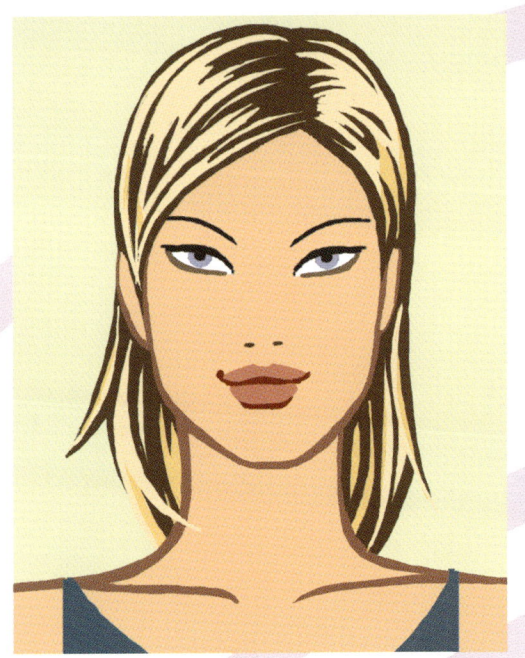
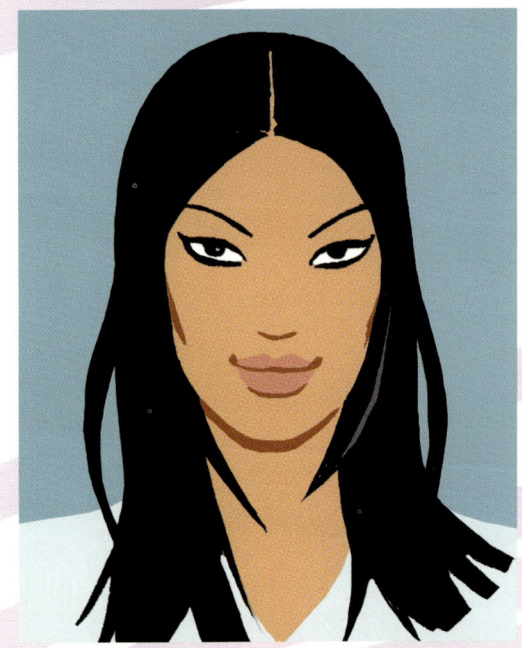

# polly

**Polly** is a city career babe – traditional, yes, but with a twist. Her double first in maths means she can tot up her buying splurges as fast as the computers at Visa. Everyone thought that Polly was as straight and reliable as her sleek blonde hair (which is actually the result of painstaking styling with straightening irons), until she announced her impetuous engagement to cyber-suitor Simon, a work colleague from New York. Simon popped the question during their luxurious holiday in the Seychelles, and an equally speedy wedding is to follow the whirlwind romance.

# jaz

**Jaz (short for Jasmine)** is your regular club bunnie. She loves all things hip, cool and girlie. Her earliest memory is of dressing up in the contents of her mother's overstuffed wardrobe – and clothes are still her greatest passion. She never takes her make-up off before bed but, with her long, glossy black hair, she always looks stunning anyway. Always the party girl, Jaz has suddenly developed a career interest she never knew she had after landing a job with Aristo PR. Combining two of her major passions, fashion and fun, she's working longer and harder than ever before and loving every minute of it.

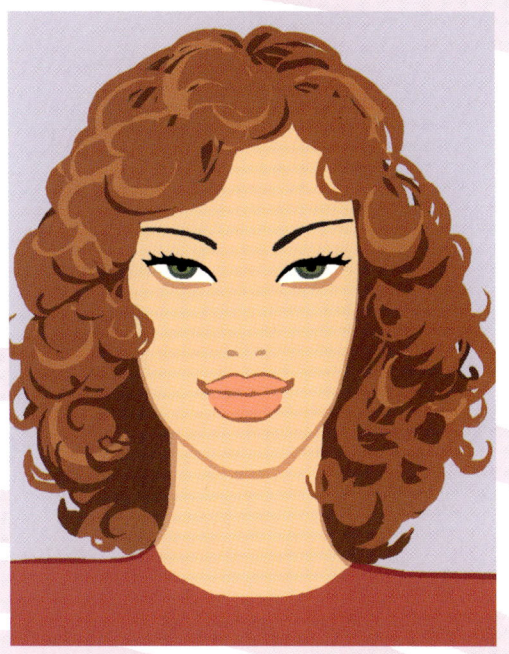 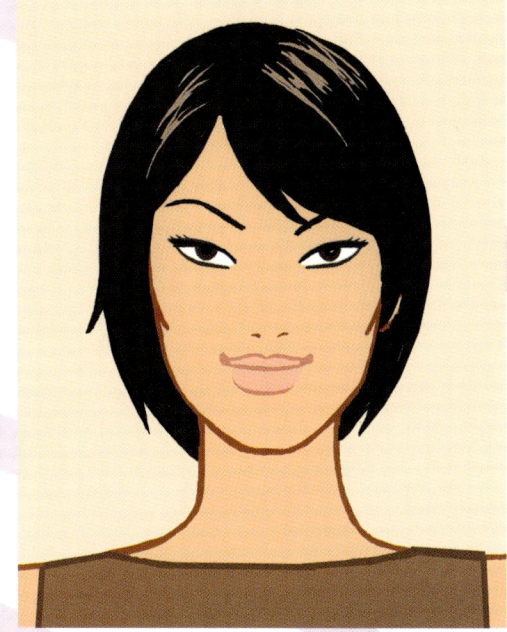

# kate

**Kate** looks like a pre-Raphaelite painting: unruly curly titian hair, milky complexion and rosy cheeks. She works as personal assistant to the marketing director of Crunch biscuits, where she feels unappreciated and underused. A recent two-week break at a yoga retreat in India has helped her to gain a new perspective on her life. She's thinking of making big changes, but so far that has only meant giving up her unrequited crush on her boss and abandoning the 'power bob' that did nothing to enhance her image at work. But she's determined not to give up her new-found confidence in herself.

# laura

**Laura** is a tomboy: lean and androgynous with a short crop. Her uniform is urban cool – more combats and trainers than pencil skirts and kitten heels. She loves to work out and applies the same intensity and dedication to her career as a TV researcher. Much to everyone's surprise (including her own), she's recently redefined her image, experimenting with a softer, more feminine look – and it seems to have paid off. She's finally won the affections of her long-term crush, John, an assistant TV producer, and now her priorities are changing.

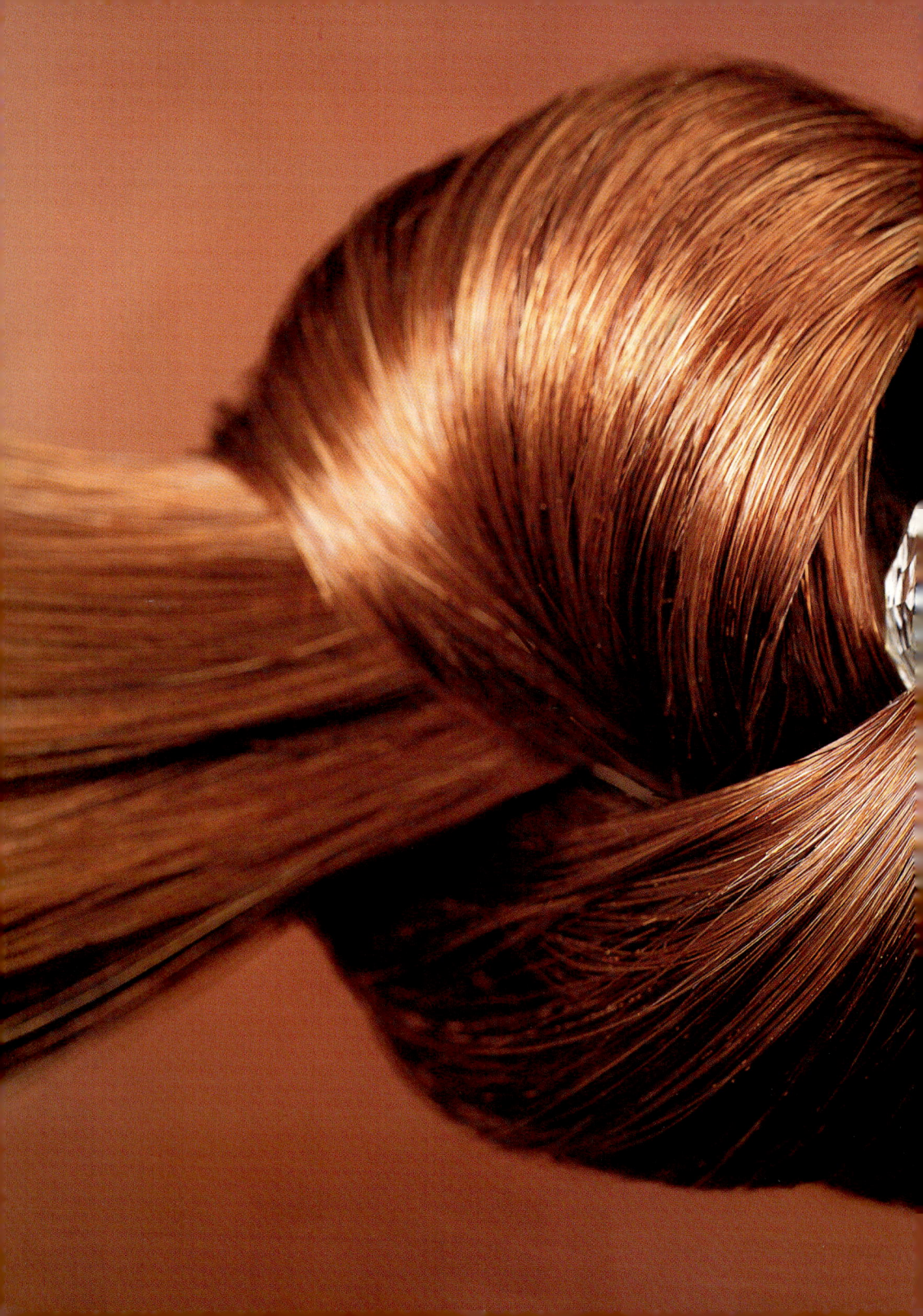

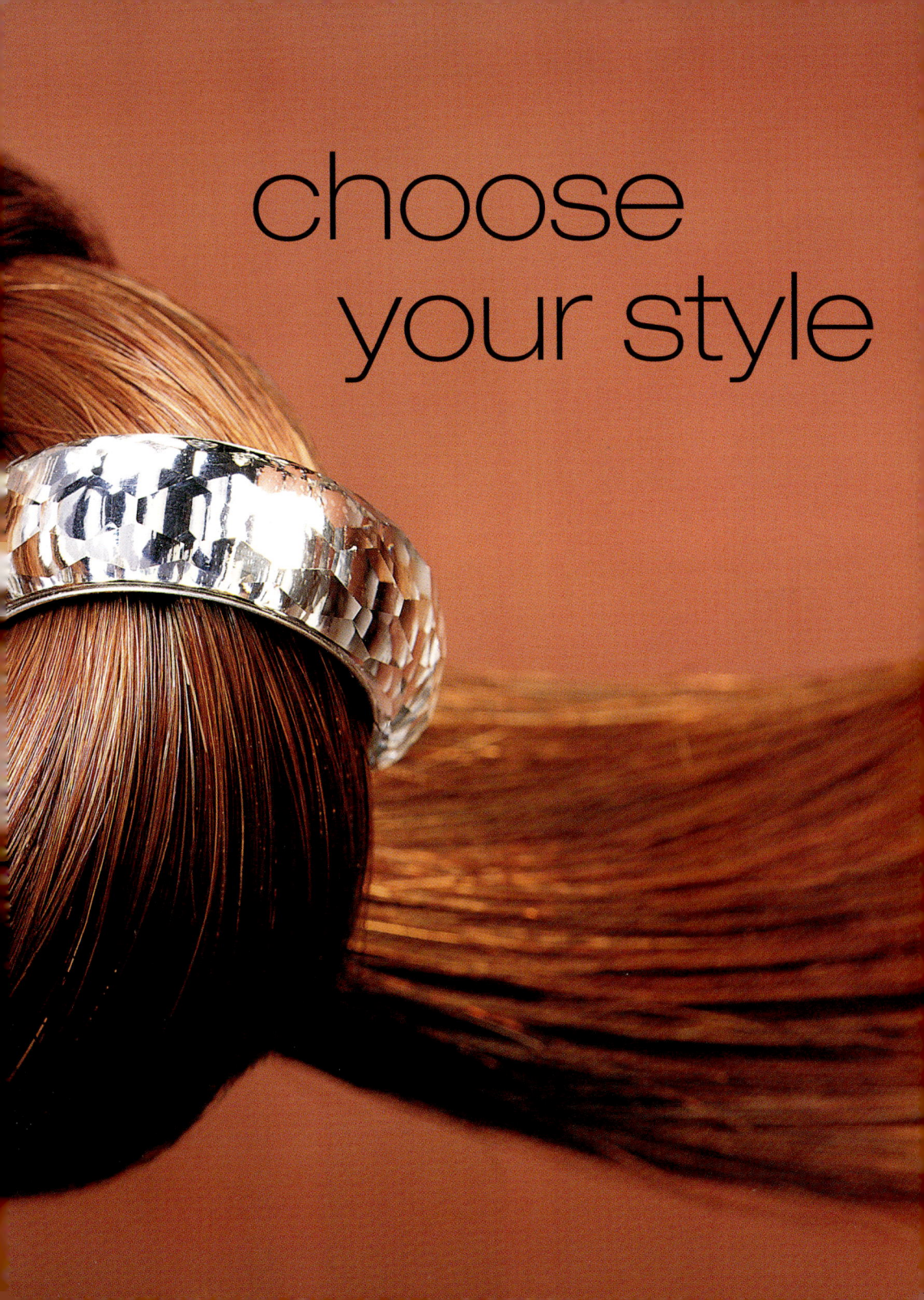

# the girls digest polly's big news

'**I think I need a drink**,' said Chrissie, the confirmed bachelorette of the group, in the light of Polly's announcement. (Chrissie had come over from New York to stay with the girls for a month, but now seemed to be a permanent fixture in the house.)
'Luckily, we have some Champagne,' beamed Polly, who couldn't contain her obvious glee. Jaz, Laura and Kate silently exchanged stunned glances, while they tried to take in the alarming fact that aliens may have abducted and replaced their dear friend, sensible 'perfect' Polly. At last, incurably romantic Kate threw her arms around Polly.
'Oh, I just knew it! This is so fabulous, you must be thrilled!' she squealed excitedly.

Laura, Polly's best friend from Manchester, was a little less enthusiastic. 'But, Polly, you've only known Simon for a few months, how can you be sure?' she asked, frowning. Polly had known that Laura would try to be the voice of reason. Even her own budding love affair with her long-term object of desire, John, didn't seem to have softened her stoic tomboy nature.
'Look, I know you're only concerned for me,' Polly said, flopping down onto the sofa next to Laura and taking her hand, 'but I know this is the right thing.' She smiled happily. 'We love each other. He's funny and kind, and he treats me really well.' (This was a veiled reference to Polly's ex-boyfriend Harry, a nice but lazy banker, who had been more interested in his bank balance than in Polly.)

'Well I think it's really wonderful,' gushed Kate, tossing her head of wild red curls defiantly. This was unlike the normally shy Kate, who could usually be relied upon for a rather cautious response. Chrissie eyed her from head to toe, taking in her smooth honey-coloured skin and her surprisingly svelte, toned thighs, revealed to their advantage by her cut-off denims. (At times, Kate had been known to overindulge in the broken rejects from her workplace, Crunch Biscuits.) To top it off, she had allowed her hair to revert to its naturally curly state, and it was made even prettier by a smattering of sun-kissed golden highlights. Chrissie, as resident glamour puss, was not amused.
'It's not like you to be so excitable, Kate. You didn't have a holiday romance, too, did you?' she purred, knowing full well about Kate's unrequited obsession with her boss, marketing director Matthew.
But Kate remained unruffled, purring back, 'Oh, this isn't about me, Chrissie, this is about Pol.' Chrissie bit back her fury – why did she feel so angry?

Polly turned to Jaz, who was the only one of her friends who had yet to express an opinion.
'Well, what do you think?' She enquired nervously.
'I think you're not taking this seriously enough at all,' Jaz responded sternly. 'Don't you realize, Polly,' she continued, her smile spreading as she caught the look on Polly's crestfallen face, 'that this is the most important dress you're ever going to buy?'

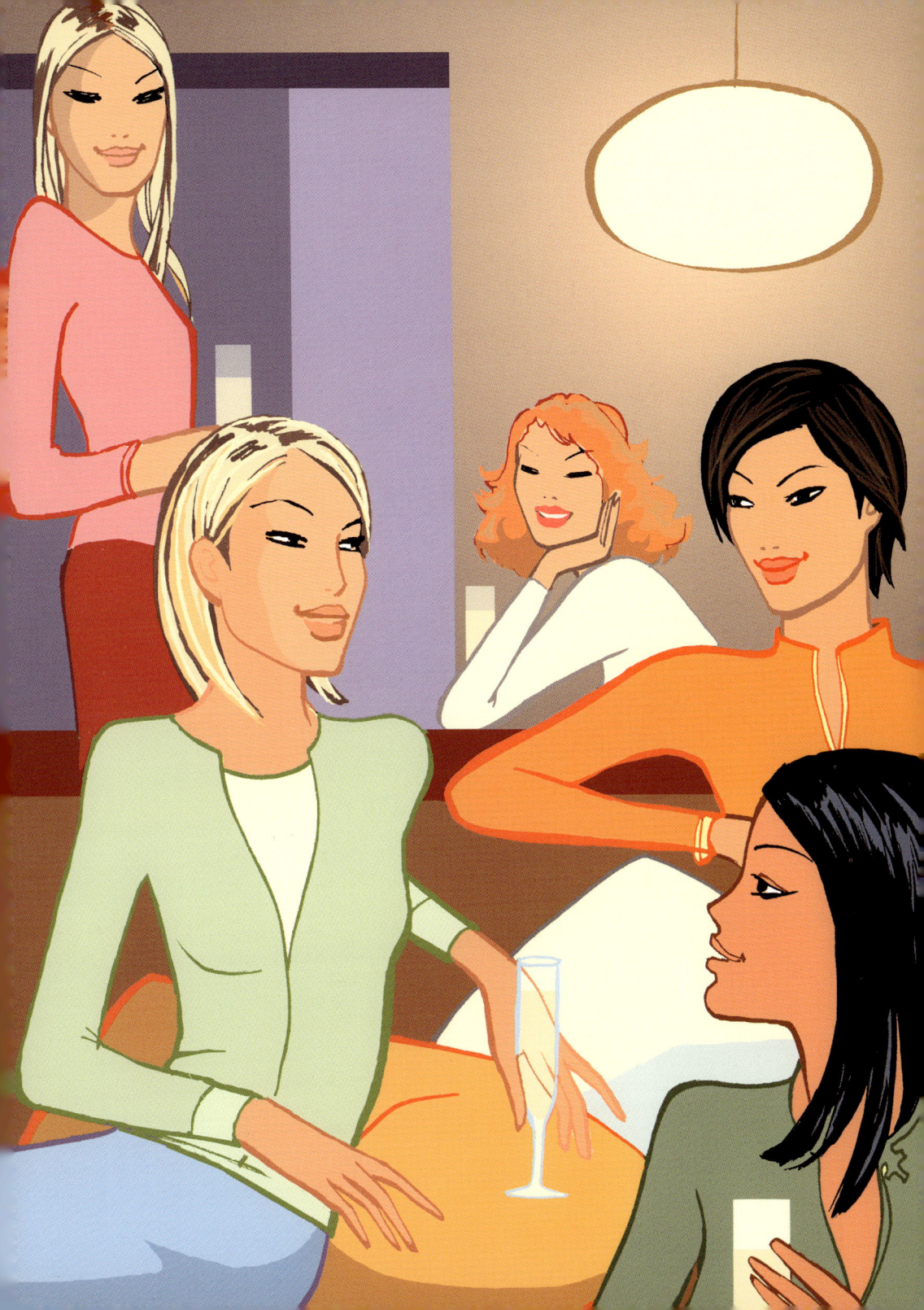

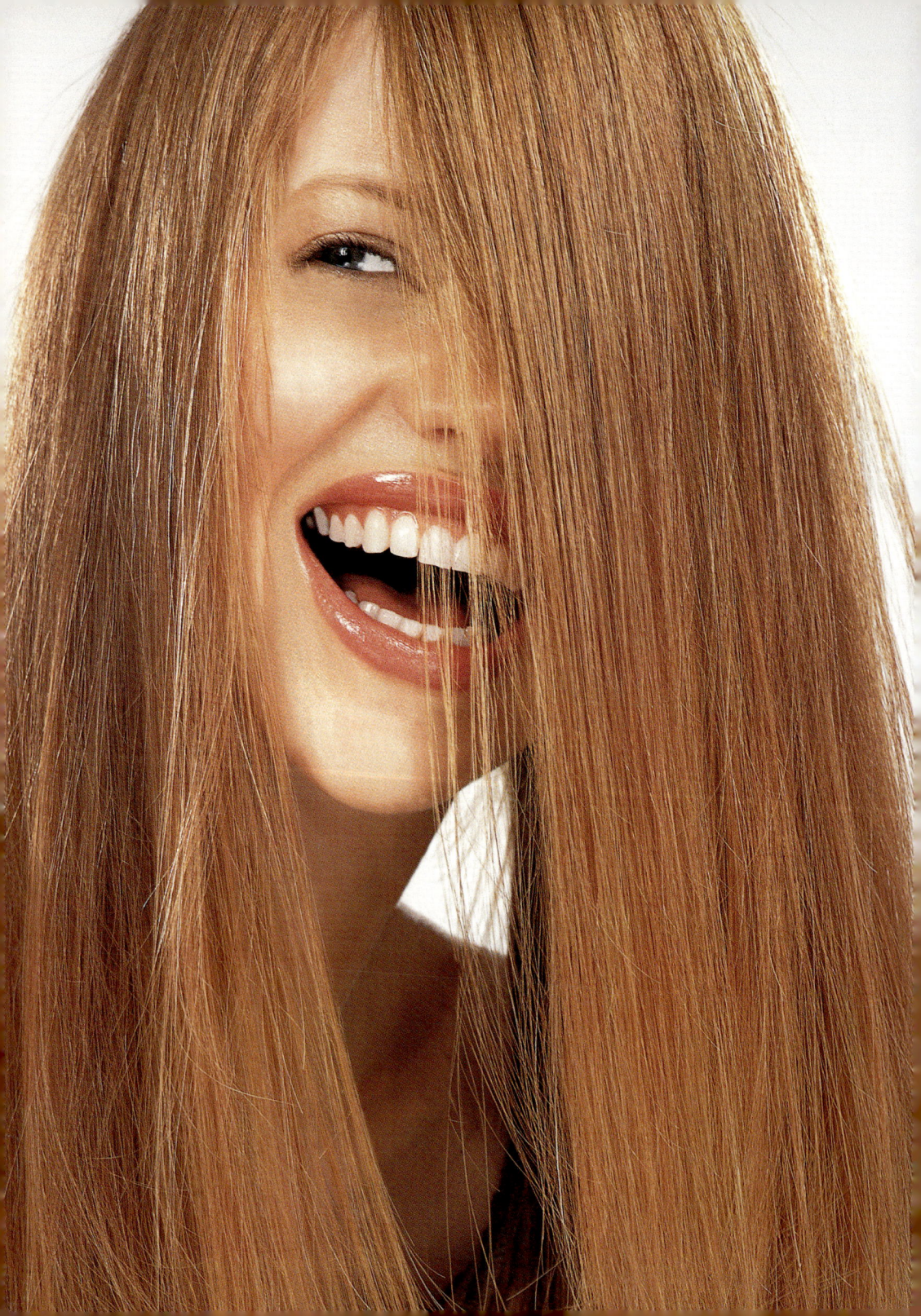

# finding a look

Forget everything you know about what suits you. Whether you live in kitten heels and pretty cardigans or trainers and denim, the chances are that the way you want to look on your wedding day will be completely unrelated to the way you look in your everyday life. And every variable will affect the hairstyle that you choose. Start by considering the following few elements.

## dress style

Have you envisaged yourself in something simple and floaty or a huge, structured confection that would be the envy of Cinderella? The way you imagine your dress to be and what style actually suits you may be two entirely different things, so take a close friend or family member shopping with you, and try on lots of different styles. You will be surprised.

## body shape and height

We are all shaped differently, and the satin bias-cut dress of our dreams might not have been part of Mother Nature's plan when she made us. As a result, you may look fabulous enhancing your tiny waist with a fitted bodice and hiding your less tiny hips under a full skirt. This means you may need a hairstyle with more body or height to create a balanced silhouette.

## neckline

Your hairstyle and dress need to work together. A low scooping neckline can look wonderfully romantic with loose tendrils of hair, whereas a chic bob with a sleek slash neck is exceptionally elegant. If you have a low back on your dress, you can draw attention to this feature by wearing your hair swept up and away from your neck. Take a photograph or sketch of your dress with you to the hairdresser's so you can consider which hairstyles will make the most of its features.

## tiaras and veils

Although it is not uncommon to have both a tiara and a veil, most brides choose to wear either one or the other. And, as weddings have become more informal, a few simple flowers dotted through the hair are also a popular alternative to both of these options. A long veil or heavy tiara will need to be held securely in place, and this will influence your choice of hairstyle. If you can, take your tiara (or at least a photograph of it) with you when you go for a consultation with your hairdresser, so that he or she can work out exactly what will need to be done on that count.

## face shape

You probably know what suits you by now, and this is not usually the time that women opt for a drastic change of look. (It's nice if he recognizes you when you're walking down the aisle.) However, unless you are a very high-maintenance girl and do your weekly shop wearing a tiara, you probably won't know how it affects the proportions of your face. A petite heart-shaped face may look better with a simple beaded tiara, rather than drowned by a grand crown and full veil. So it's back to dressing up – try on lots of styles and see if your reality matches your fantasy.

## jewellery

One of the 'Something old, something new ...' categories is often fulfilled with jewellery. So, whether you choose a string of antique pearls from your grandmother or a funky, dramatic choker from one of your bridesmaids, it needs consideration at this stage, too. A tiara, veil, earrings, choker and high collar can quickly become very fussy. Don't let your look become cluttered – less is always more (even with diamonds).

**HAIR SNIP**
WHEN CHOOSING ACCESSORIES FOR YOUR HAIR, WHETHER IT IS FRESH FLOWERS OR AN ANTIQUE BROOCH, MAKE SURE IT IS IN BALANCE WITH THE REST OF YOUR OUTFIT – SOMETIMES LESS IS MORE.

**In beauty and fashion** matters, Jaz is regarded as the oracle, so Polly invites her along to her appointment with Charles, her trusted stylist. For the last few years, he has kept her wavy locks blonder and straighter than nature ever intended them to be.

Despite her impetuous decision to get married, Polly's cautious nature has reasserted itself and she pulls from her bag a neat file of pictures from bridal magazines. At the same time, Jaz produces a jumble of catwalk photos, slides from hair shows (borrowed from Aristo PR) and pages torn out of *Gloss* magazine. Charles grins and tells the girls that they need to go back to basics. Polly's hair has a natural wave, which she usually straightens and smoothes with a glossing serum. The sun has lightened it to a uniform, creamy blonde that works well with her tan, but makes her fine hair seem thin. They agree that she should have caramel lowlights to make her hair look thicker.

Next, they look at pictures of the dress. Polly has chosen a close-fitting, full-length dress in off-white duchesse satin. Chic and elegant, it has a high neck,

## ... polly's consultation with charles

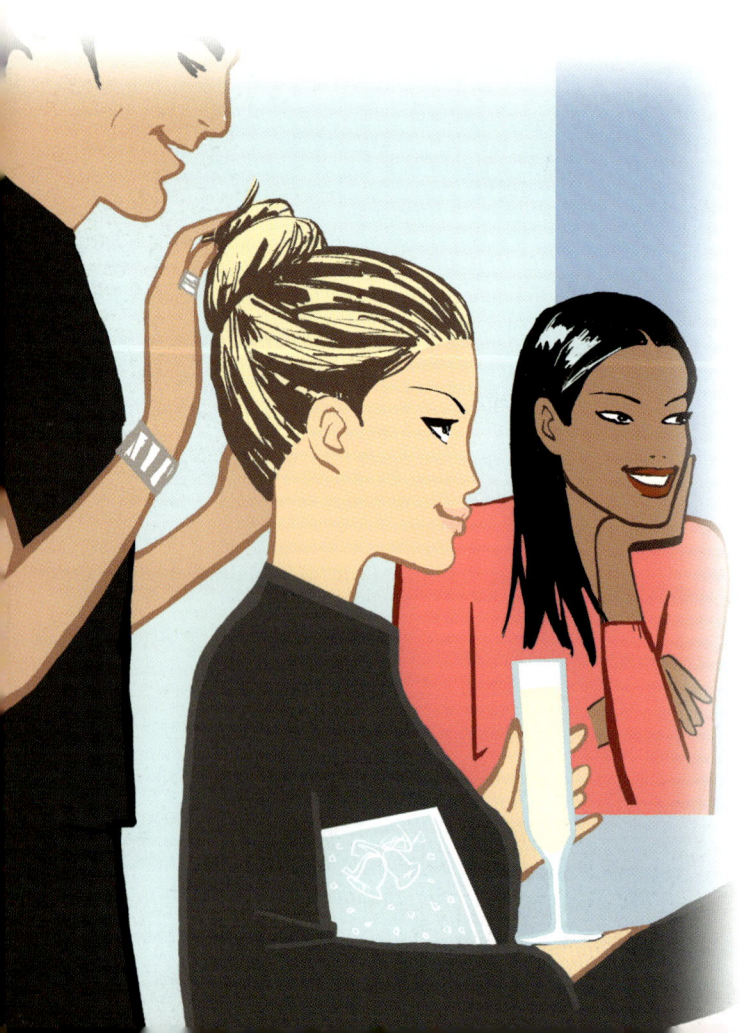

three-quarter length sleeves and a low, scooped back. For protection from the elements, she's chosen a fitted high-collar jacket. Charles believes that such a formal dress deserves a formal updo. The hair should be swept up to draw attention to the dramatic plunging dress and show off her slender, tanned back. The next consideration is the jacket, the high collar of which will skim the back of her neck. Charles thinks that to avoid looking fussy, her hairstyle must be simple and clean (which rules out Jaz's pictures of a half-up, half-down do with wispy tendrils and diamanté clips). After much wrangling (veil too much with the jacket, jewellery too fussy for the neckline), they settle on a classic chignon, with a tiara and simple diamond earrings. A slightly despondent Jaz (doesn't Polly know that matrimony is fashionable?) is cheered when Polly escorts her out of the salon, telling her it's time to select the bridesmaids' dresses.

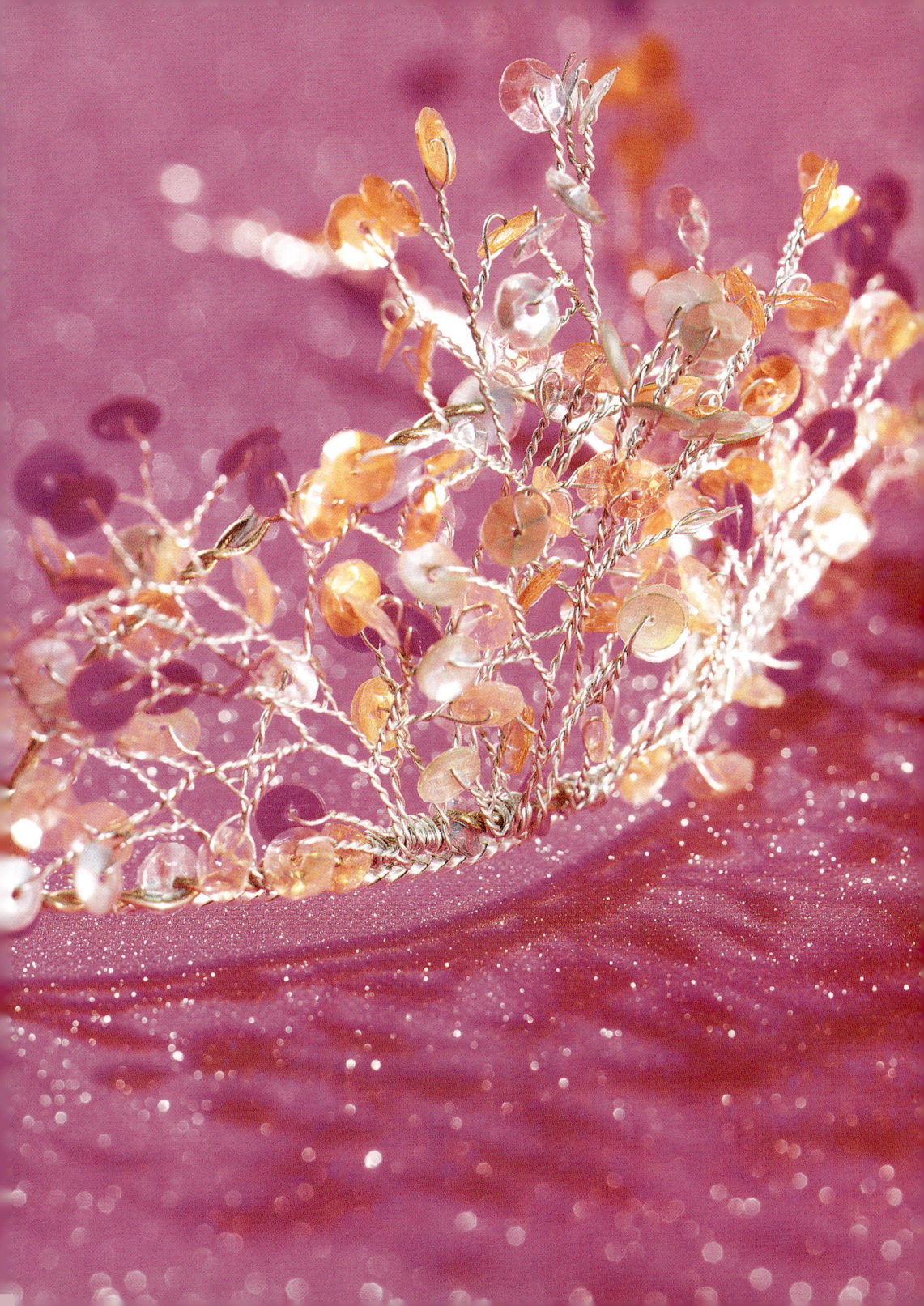

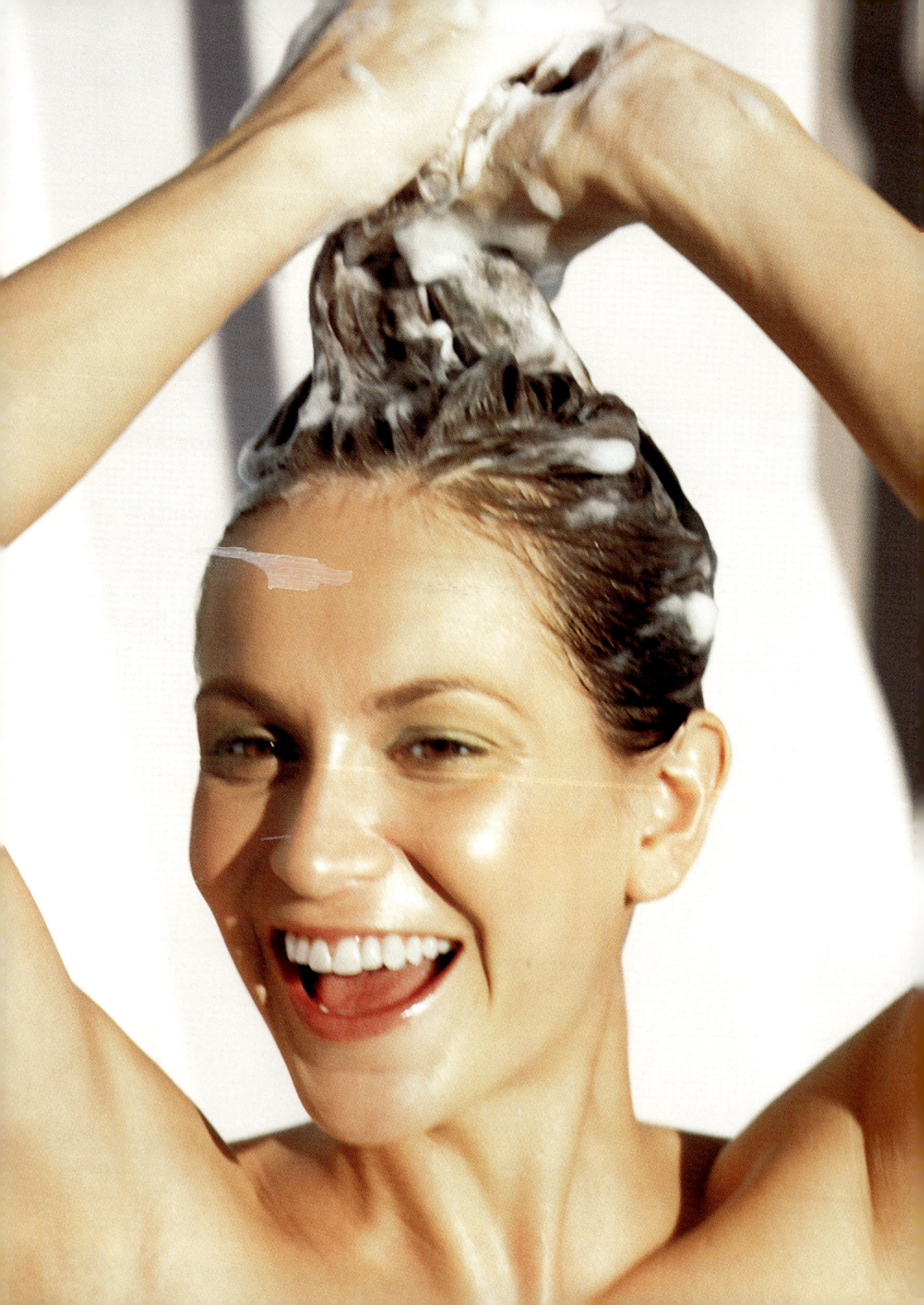

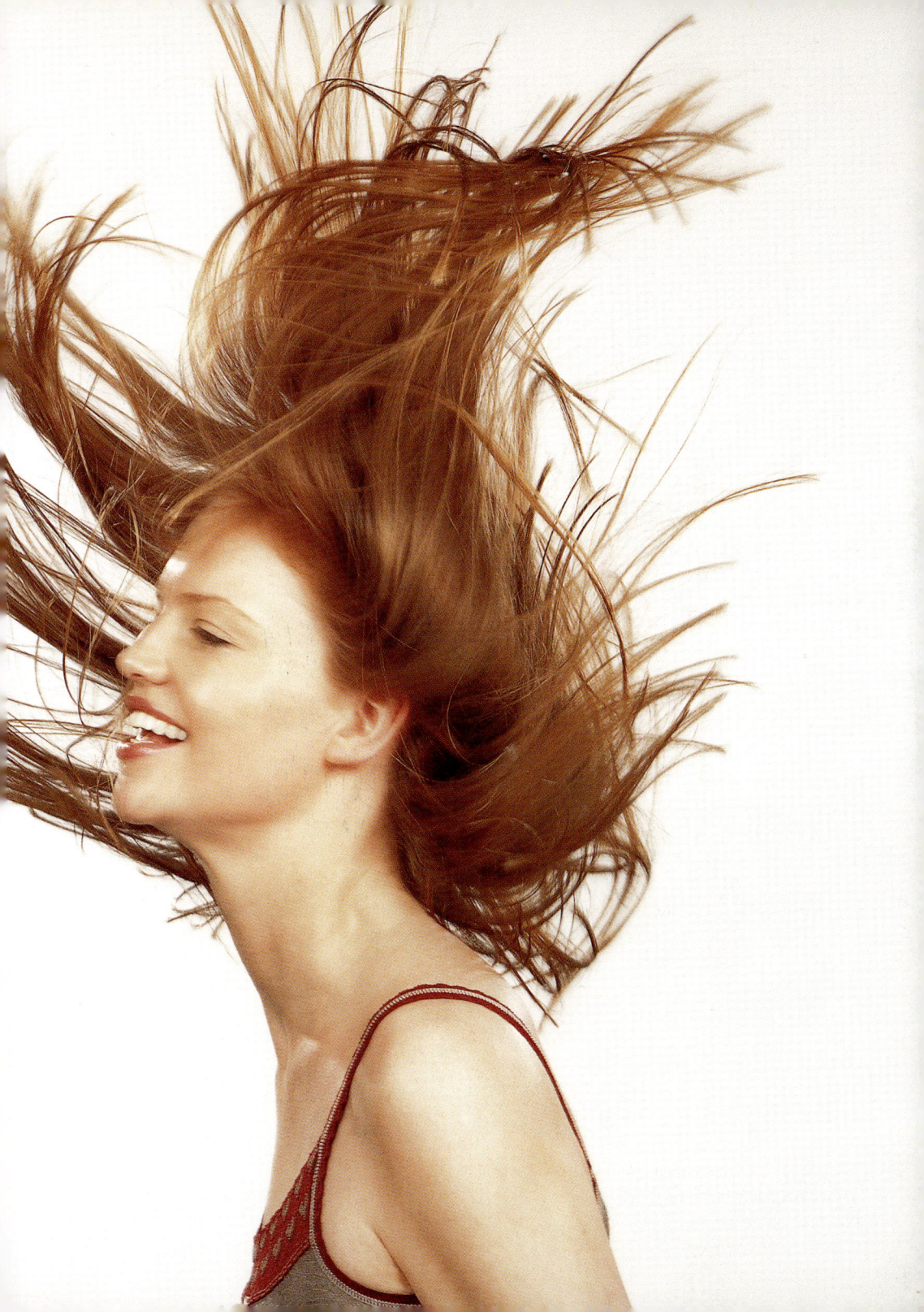

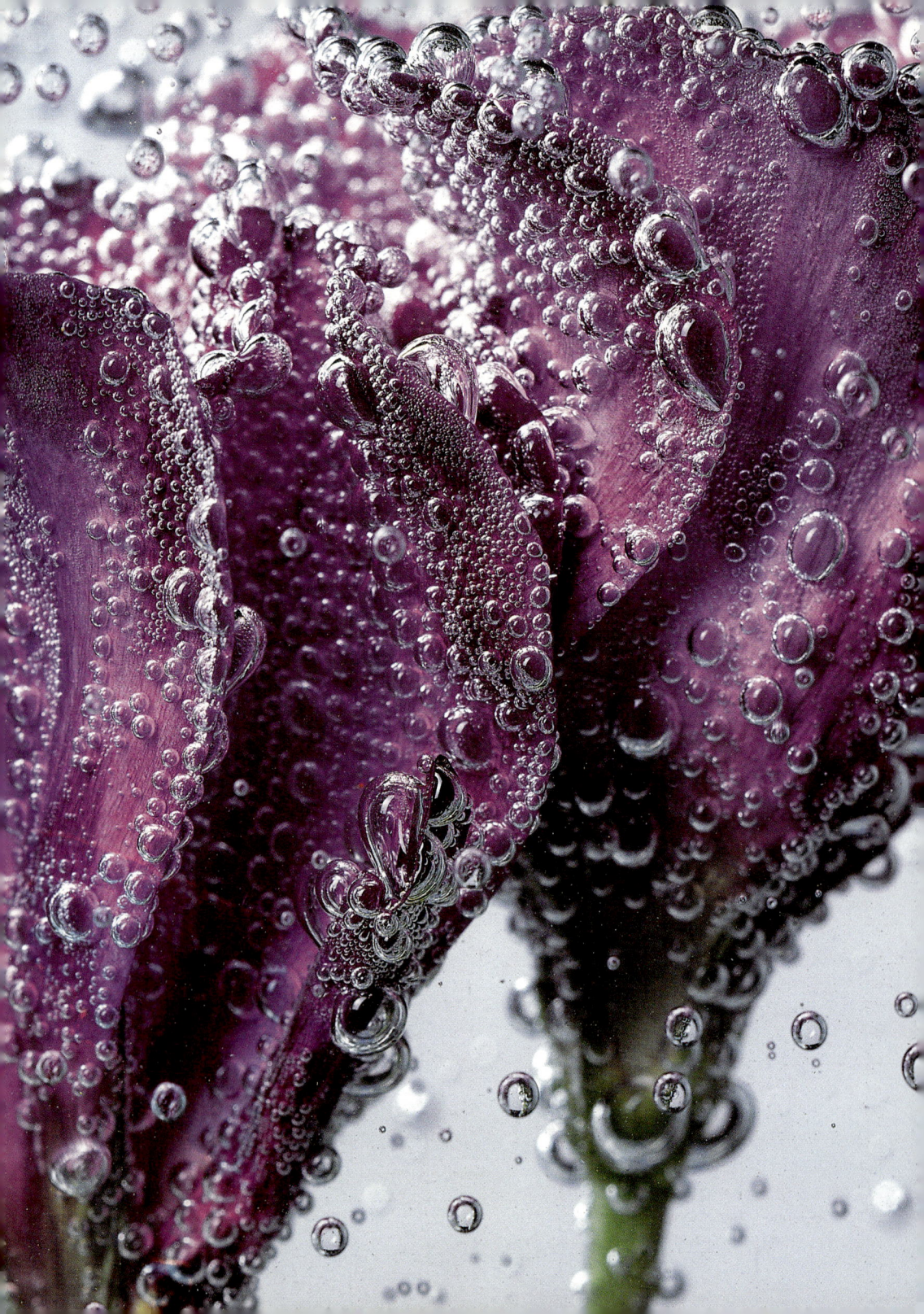

**Laura knows that** she has changed since meeting John, much more so than she'd like to admit. After spending such a long time hoping to get his attention, things are moving pretty fast. She's even had to acknowledge that her growing interest in her appearance is less to do with sharing a flat with looks-obsessed Chrissie and Jaz, and more to do with catching John's attention.

After the initial shock, Laura has become more supportive of what she considers to be Polly's impulsive decision to marry Simon – despite the fact it might leave them all homeless. It may also have something to do with flattery – Polly has asked her to be Maid of Honour (although Laura sometimes wonders whether Polly reached this decision largely because of her organizational skills, especially considering the lack of help she's had from the others with planning the hen night).

Laura's decided to see her stylist about growing her short hair, hoping that a slightly longer style will seem less severe next to Polly's sleek updo. Her hairdresser, who helped her restyle her hair earlier in the year from a low-maintenance crop to a slightly longer fringe (bangs) and light flick-outs at the nape, is thrilled to get a second chance to reinvent Laura. In two and a half months, hair will grow approximately 2.5 cm (1 1/4 inches). As Laura's current style is already beginning to grow out, her stylist suggests letting the fringe (bangs) grow out and having it cut over to one side. The rest of her hair will be allowed to grow into a sleek, slightly layered short bob – feminine, but still right for Laura's usual uniform of T-shirt and combats.

# ... laura goes for another restyle

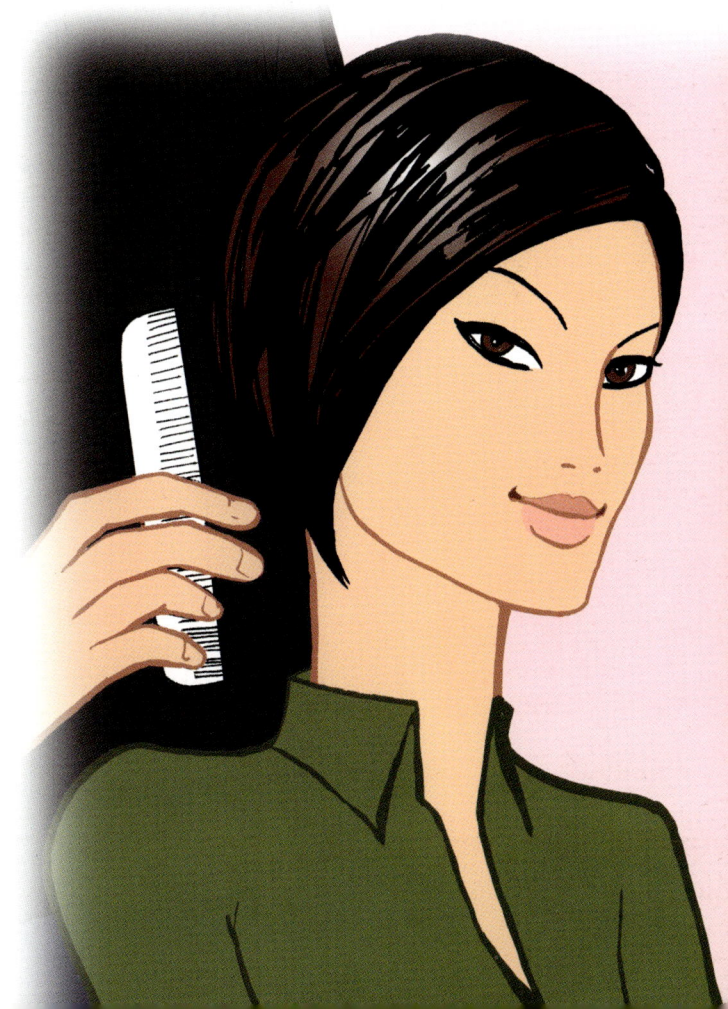

CHOOSE YOUR STYLE

# wedding wisdom

As soon as a girl accepts a proposal, everyone has an opinion. Hopefully these tips should help you keep focused on what you want.

**1** Start cheating. Don't be despondent if you think your hair doesn't naturally have the qualities you want. This is the most special of occasions and your style doesn't have to be practical or able to function in the real world – just as long as you can make it last the day. There are many tricks of the trade to help you create the illusion that you want: hairpieces can add volume, straighteners can make hair ultra-sleek and a well-placed veil can make even short hair appear long. Your hairdresser could be your greatest ally.

**2** If you are wearing a long veil, keep your hairstyle as simple as possible.

**3** Don't be tempted to go for a radical restyle – it's you he has asked to marry and it's you he wants to see at the altar.

**4** How will you get to the church? Whether it's a horse-drawn carriage or a moped, tell your stylist so that he or she can disaster-proof you!

**5** Remember to have long hair trimmed before the big day – even a couple of centimetres (an inch) of growth could make the style you have settled on impossible to achieve.

**6** Always have a full trial run with your veil and/or tiara before the big day.

**7** If you are not happy with what your hairdresser has done, you must tell them. He or she would rather start again than have it ruin your day.

**8** Your dress, veil, flowers, tiara, hair and even shoes should all create a cohesive look – give your stylist as much visual reference as you can to allow them to help you achieve that.

**9** There's no need to change hairdressers if you have a good rapport with your current one. He or she knows your hair and how to get the best from it. Do make sure, though, that they feel comfortable doing it. (Your favourite colourist, for example, may not be the person for the job!)

**10** Don't get an attack of 'wedding ringlets'. If your style is simple, don't let others bully you into a look you don't feel comfortable with just because they perceive it as being more glamorous.

**11** Short hair can look just as feminine as longer styles, and if you know that it suits you, you're better off sticking with what you've got.

**12** Some subtle highlights around the face are a great way to lift the complexion and draw attention to the face.

**13** Make sure you give plenty of notice if you want a particular stylist to do your hair on the morning of the wedding.

**14** Using every styling product on the market to try and keep your hair in place will only make it look dirty and weighed down. Select products well and have a trial run to see how much you really need.

**15** Work with your hair type if you can – will your long, poker-straight hair really stay in curls all day?

**16** Take a camera to the hairdresser's with you. You will be surprised how something that looks good in real life doesn't always look great in photographs. This will also give you some reference material to show to your family and friends.

**17** You must start planning your hairstyle approximately three months in advance. This means that you will have the time to get your hair into top condition, with two or three conditioning treatments at your salon, and have two trial runs of the actual style. Having trial runs will make sure you get the style just right so that you feel more positive about the day.

CHOOSE YOUR STYLE

# countdown

In an ideal world, brides would begin thinking about their haircare regime at least nine months before the wedding. This would allow ample time to improve the condition of the hair with treatments and any necessary changes to diet and lifestyle before even choosing a hairstyle. This is especially important if you suffer from alopecia (hair loss) or seborheic dermatitis (a condition that results in a flaky scalp); these are often caused by a dietry deficiency and can be treated by a trichologist (see page 17). Likewise, if your hair is in poor condition due to chemical processing or overstyling, make an appointment to see your hairdresser as soon as you can to allow time for them to implement an effective treatment programme.

Ultimately, your hairdo and the accessories you choose should reflect your style and personality in the same way as your choice of dress. So, while it is a good idea to gather inspiration from magazines, don't force yourself to adopt a look that is not really 'you'. Try not to change yourself too much, but make the most of what you've got and maximize your good points. Always take a photo or sketch of your dress and a swatch of fabric to your first hair consultation and ask your hairdresser's advice on accessories and flowers. You might like to try out a few different hairstyles before settling on the right one, and always have a full trial run – complete with accessories, veil and tiara – in advance of the big day. Take someone with you whose advice you trust for an honest second opinion. Use the table below to help you plan ahead.

## pre-wedding hair tips

Are you using the right haircare products for your hair type? For example, if your hair is fine and lank, this may be due to your conditioner being too heavy. Assess the condition of your hair and look at your current haircare regime.

Collect pictures for your scrapbook of hairstyles and colours that you like from all sources, not just from wedding magazines.

Do take polaroids of your hair rehearsals – otherwise it will be impossible for you or your hairdresser to remember every detail.

Even if results seem slow to emerge, stick with your treatment plan. The effects are cumulative and the end result will be worth it.

In the period leading up to your wedding, try and give your hair a break from intensive styling methods whenever possible.

Florists can provide blooms all year round now, but find out which will be in season on the big day. It's a sweet reminder of your wedding to see the flowers you wore in your hair in bloom for your anniversary in years to come.

| 6 months | 5 months | 4 months | 3 months | 2 months | 1 month |
|---|---|---|---|---|---|
| See your hairdresser to discuss your plans and book in all your appointments. | Experiment with various colour options so you can achieve the optimum look. | Collect a scrapbook of style options and discuss these with your stylist. | Begin weekly conditioning treatments. | Order the flowers for your hair. Have your first trial run at the salon. | Have a second trial run with your veil/tiara. Reconfirm your final cut and colour. |

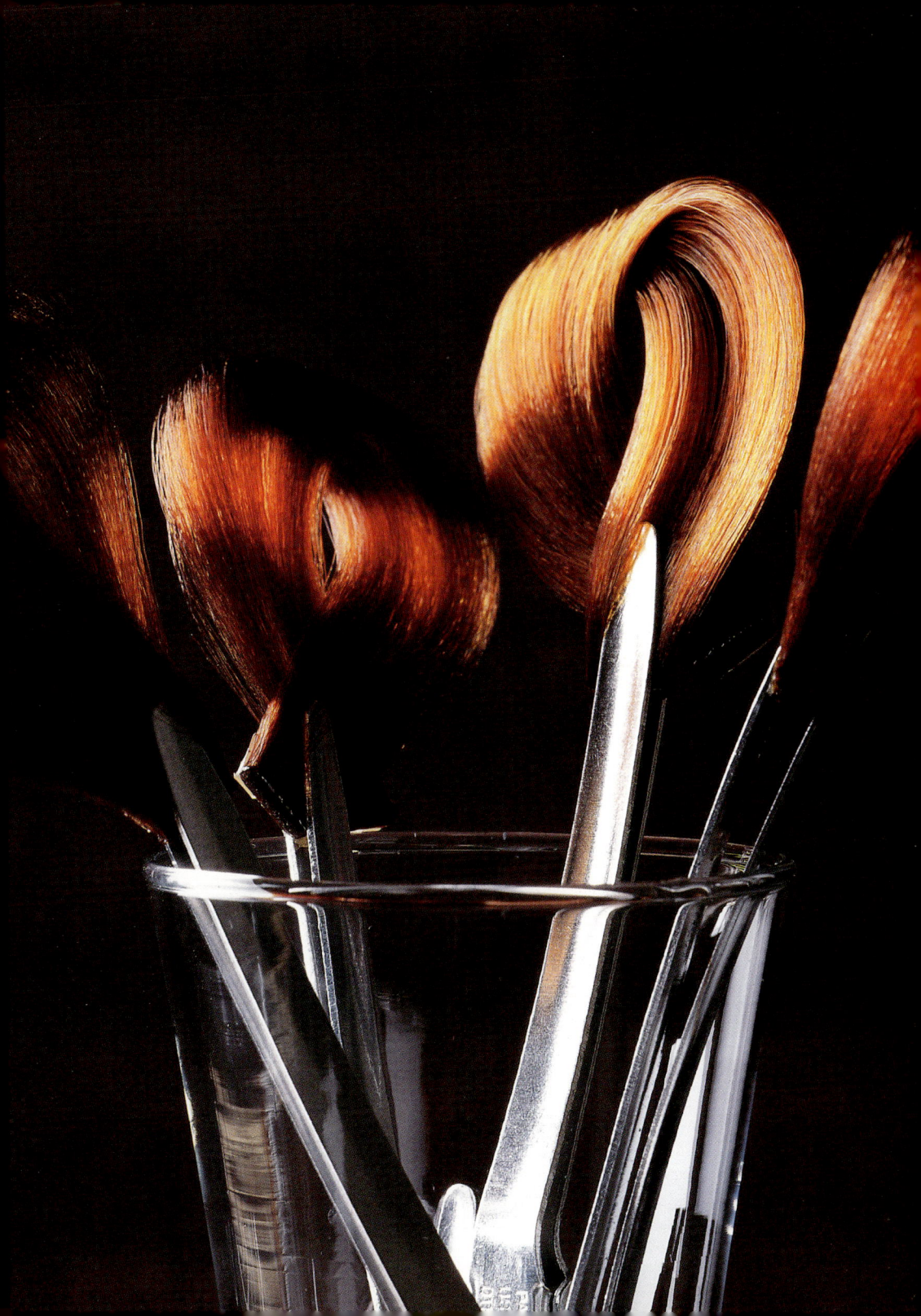

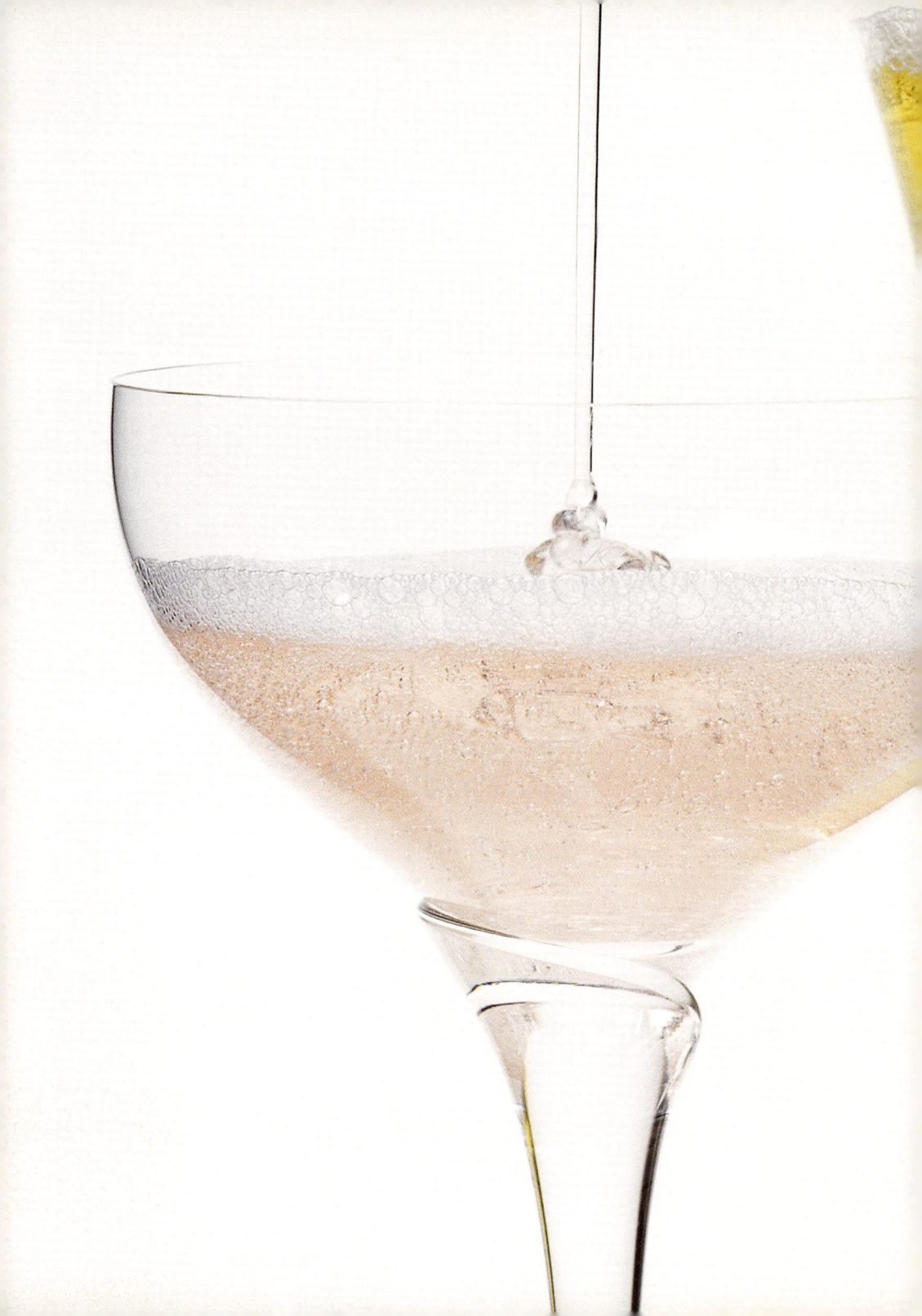

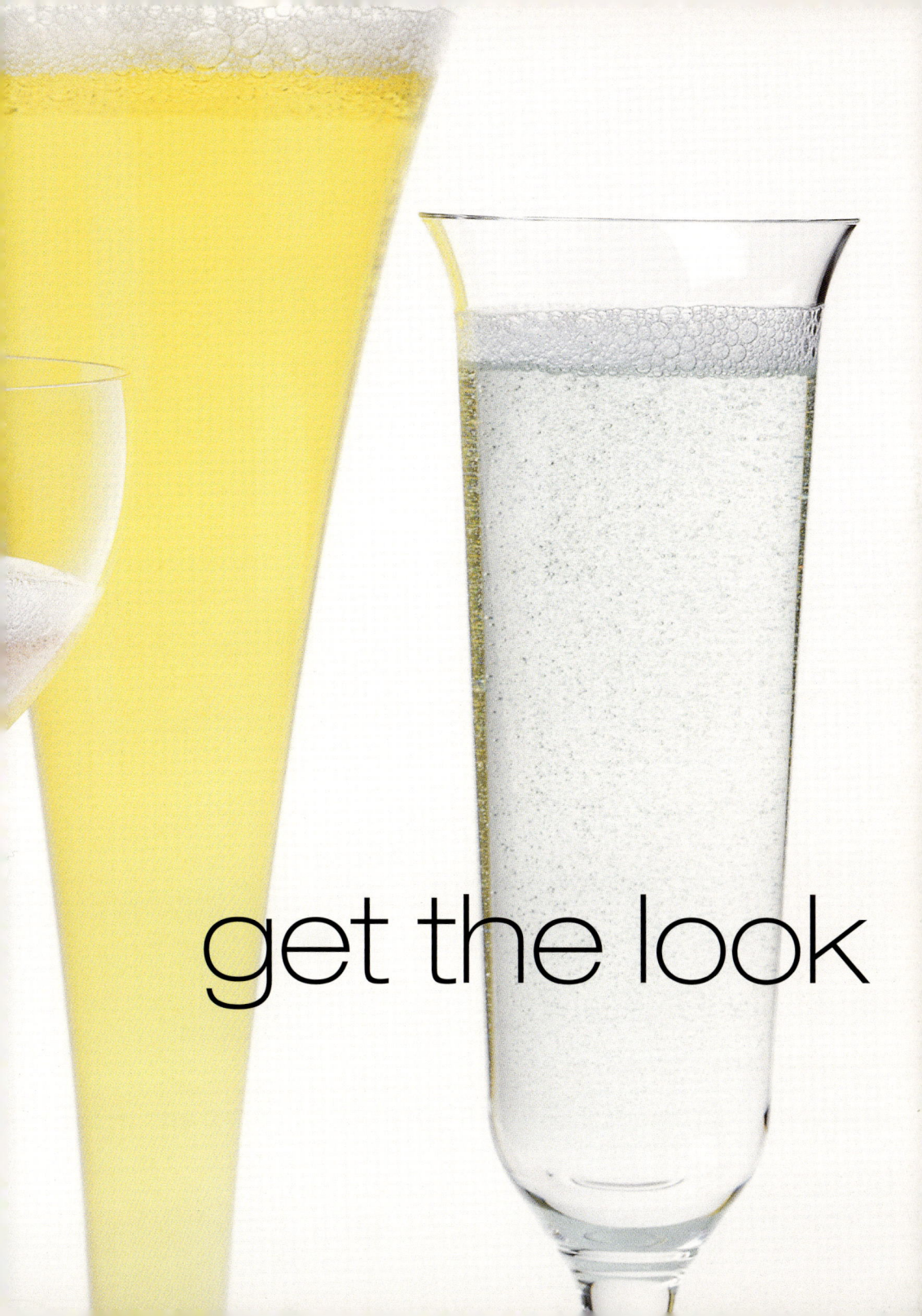
get the look

# wedding fever hits the house

**Every surface of Polly's formerly** immaculate house was covered with wedding magazines, invitations, lists and scraps of fabric.

'I would have thought,' said Chrissie, pinching a piece of Laura's toast and munching it cautiously through her regular Saturday morning face pack, 'that you would have approached this wedding with your usual degree of organization.' Laura and Kate exchanged glances. Chrissie was becoming unbearable, always ready with a sharp word or criticism.

'You try organizing a wedding in only two months,' sighed Polly, oblivious of Chrissie's critical tone. 'Now, let's get on with the business in hand – your outfits.'

Jaz started to wriggle on her chair, never more excited than when talking about clothes. 'Well, girls, we chose the fabric last week and I think you are just going to love it!' she squealed. The girls held their breath collectively – why on earth was Polly letting Jaz choose their dresses? Did she really want them tripping down the aisle in leopard skin and neon fishnets? Jaz pulled out two swatches of fabric, silk georgette in pale pink and lilac. So far, so elegant. Surely there had to be a catch.

'We thought,' said Polly, enjoying their surprise, 'or rather Jaz did, that these two colours would suit all your hair and skin tones.'

'And,' added Jaz excitedly, 'that we would have each dress in the colour you choose with a contrasting detail. For example, Laura, with your dark hair, you'd look lovely in lilac with a spilt revealing the pink; and Kate, you'd suit pink with a draped neck lined with lilac.'

Chrissie was impressed and slightly annoyed – maybe Jaz knew more about fashion than just trends. 'So we don't all have to look the same?' she asked – she hated the thought of resembling anyone else.

'Well, within reason,' cautioned Polly. 'But since you're all different shapes, as well as such different characters, it makes sense to let you all have an input and make the most of your best features.'

'And what about our hair?' asked Chrissie, who had long believed that her straight, blonde, shiny hair was the secret to all her powers. She had been praying that Polly wouldn't expect her to hide it all away in a childish corn plait or, worse, an attack of dreaded 'wedding ringlets'.

'Well, I want you all to incorporate some little pink roses into your style in some way, but how is entirely up to you. Just nothing too crazy,' Polly said, eyeing Jaz's latest tie-dyed style.

'What about your hair?' asked Kate. Polly beamed, 'Well, I'm not giving too much away, but I saw Charles last week and we have a plan – I'm getting it cut and coloured the week before, and in the mean time I'm having treatments every two weeks to improve the condition.' She paused to pop a slab of buttery, white muffin into her mouth. Kate looked startled.

'But don't you know that what you put into your body is just as influential to your hair's condition as what you treat it with externally? By the time you get married all the stress of the planning, late nights and takeaways will start showing in your hair.' Polly sipped her coffee guiltily – Kate was right, she had been pushing herself extra hard at work to get things finished so she could go on a long honeymoon. Simon was still in New York, so all the planning was left mainly to her. On top of that, she still hadn't told the girls that she wasn't moving to New York to be with Simon, but that he would be transferring to London. That meant that they would want the house for themselves – and the girls would have to move out. She was definitely a woman under pressure.

'There's nothing like a convert for giving unsolicited advice,' said Chrissie, referring to Kate's recent transformation from biscuit-muncher to abs-cruncher. Sensing Kate's and Chrissie's rivalry, Laura stepped in. 'Don't forget, everyone, that I expect you all to be ready to hit the bars running next Saturday for one of Polly's last nights of freedom.' She wrapped an arm around each of the girls' shoulders, 'and I expect all of Polly's friends to be very friendly.'

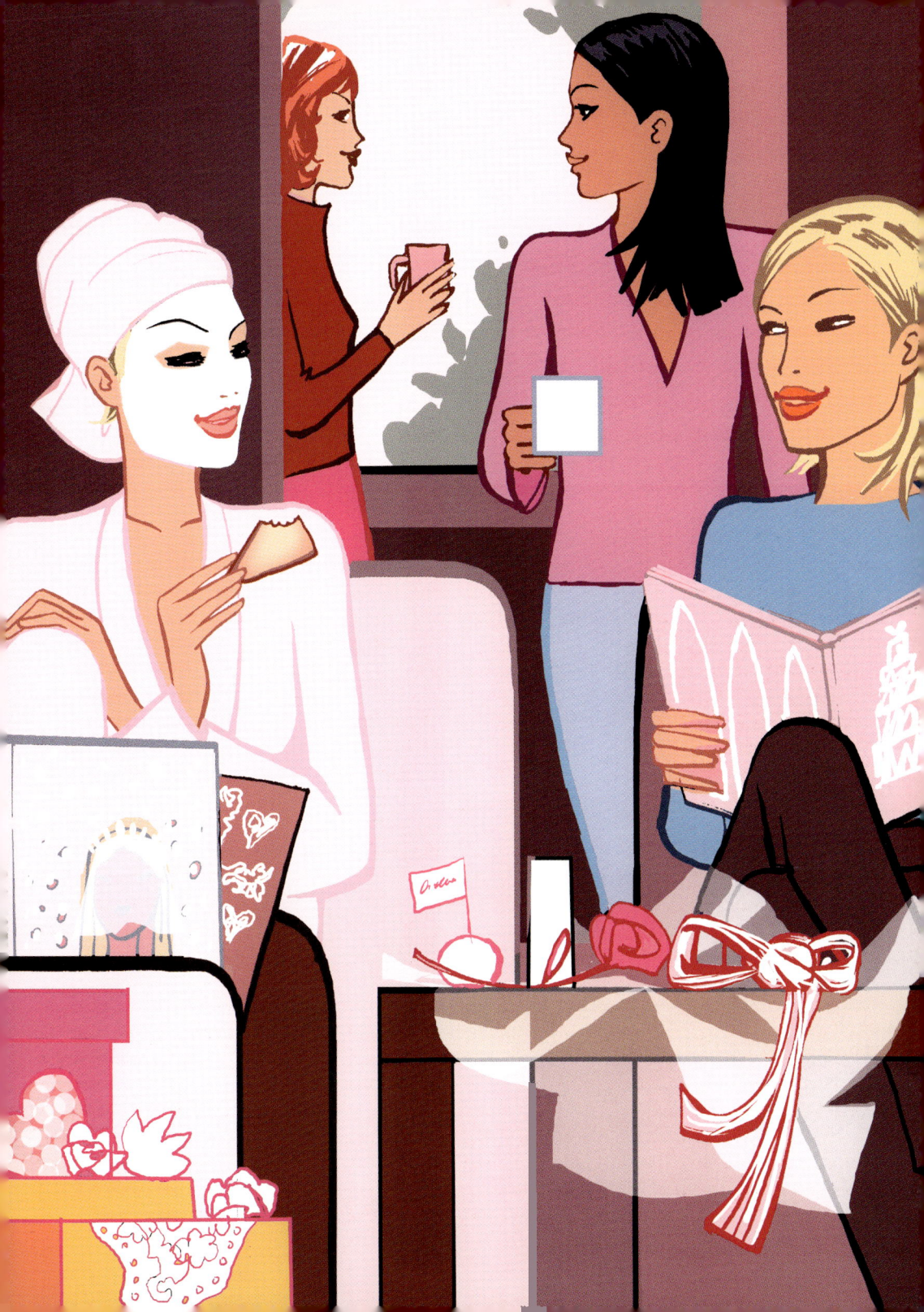

# boho vintage

This girl is never happier than when rummaging through antique shops and flea markets, searching for vintage tea dresses, silk gloves and beaded purses. At the end of her bed she keeps an old pine trunk, overflowing with diaphanous slips, pretty scraps of antique lace and crochet, and romantic Victorian nightgowns. For her wedding day, she'd team a snugly fitting Edwardian bodice with a full tulle skirt, and wear a romantic amethyst choker at her throat.

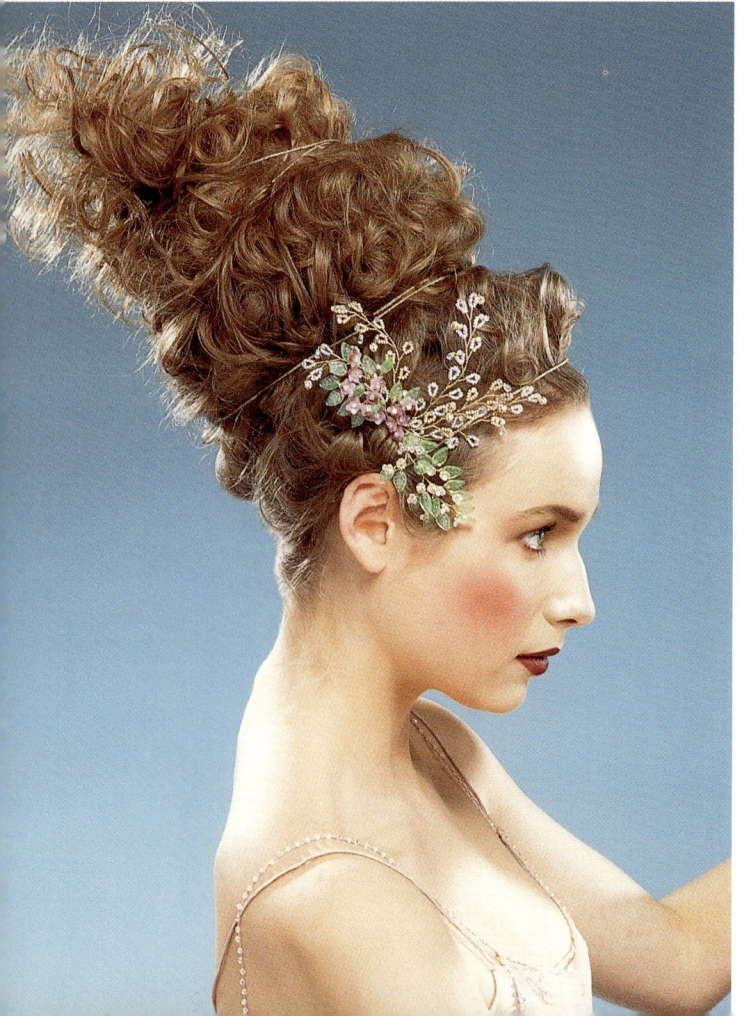

## hair solutions

If you have long hair, you could opt for a half-up, half-down do, with your hair half obscuring your crown, but with delicate tendrils framing your face. Mid-length hair can create the illusion of length when it is pulled back under a two-tier lace veil. Short hair can be softened with light-hold wax and decorated with beaded clips or ornaments, such as butterflies.

**LEFT AND RIGHT**

The hair is tonged using a light blow-dry spray to give flexibility and movement. Three bun rings are pinned together and placed on the crown of the head. The hair is wrapped around the rings, pinned securely in place and finished with firm-hold hairspray. A natural-coloured cord is wound around the hair and fastened behind the ear. If you want to dress the hair further, add an ornate hair pin on one side of the head, and hold it in place using fine pins.

**OVERLEAF**

To create this romantic look, you can employ either the classic technique of plaiting damp hair and leaving it to dry before unravelling the plaits, or the modern technique of using a hot waving iron. Use a glossing spray to finish and simply dress the style with a fine necklace or hair ornament pinned around the forehead.

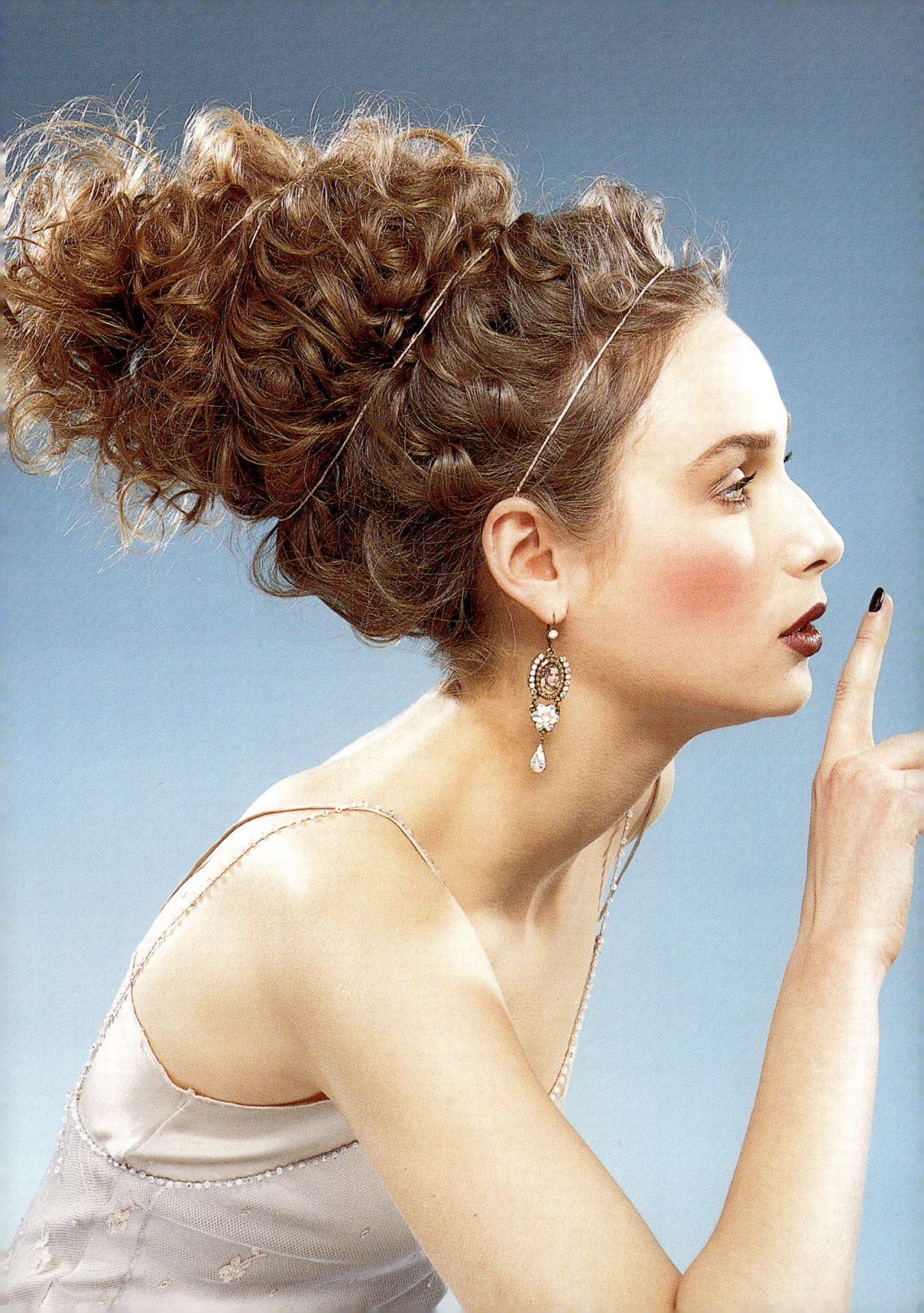

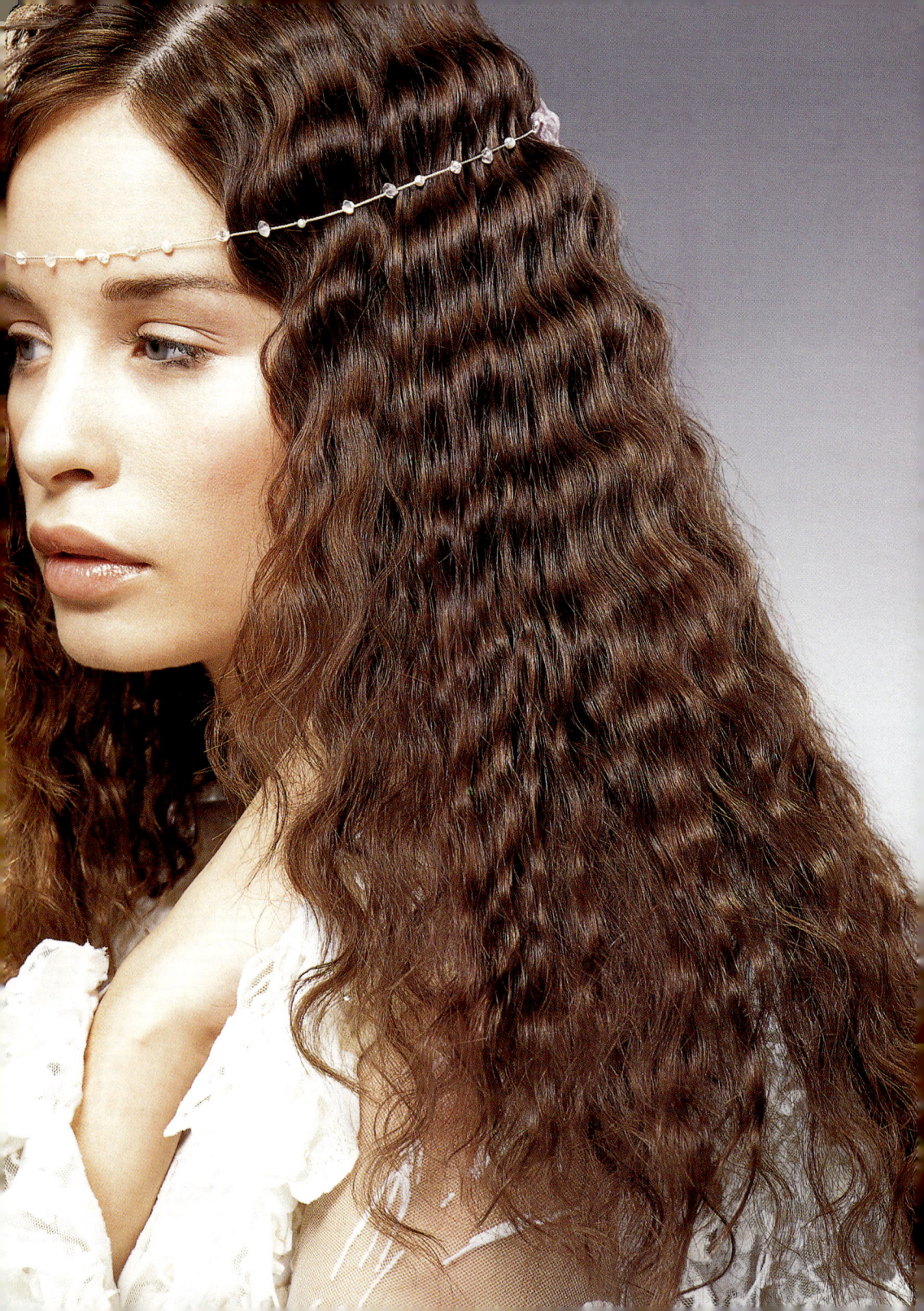

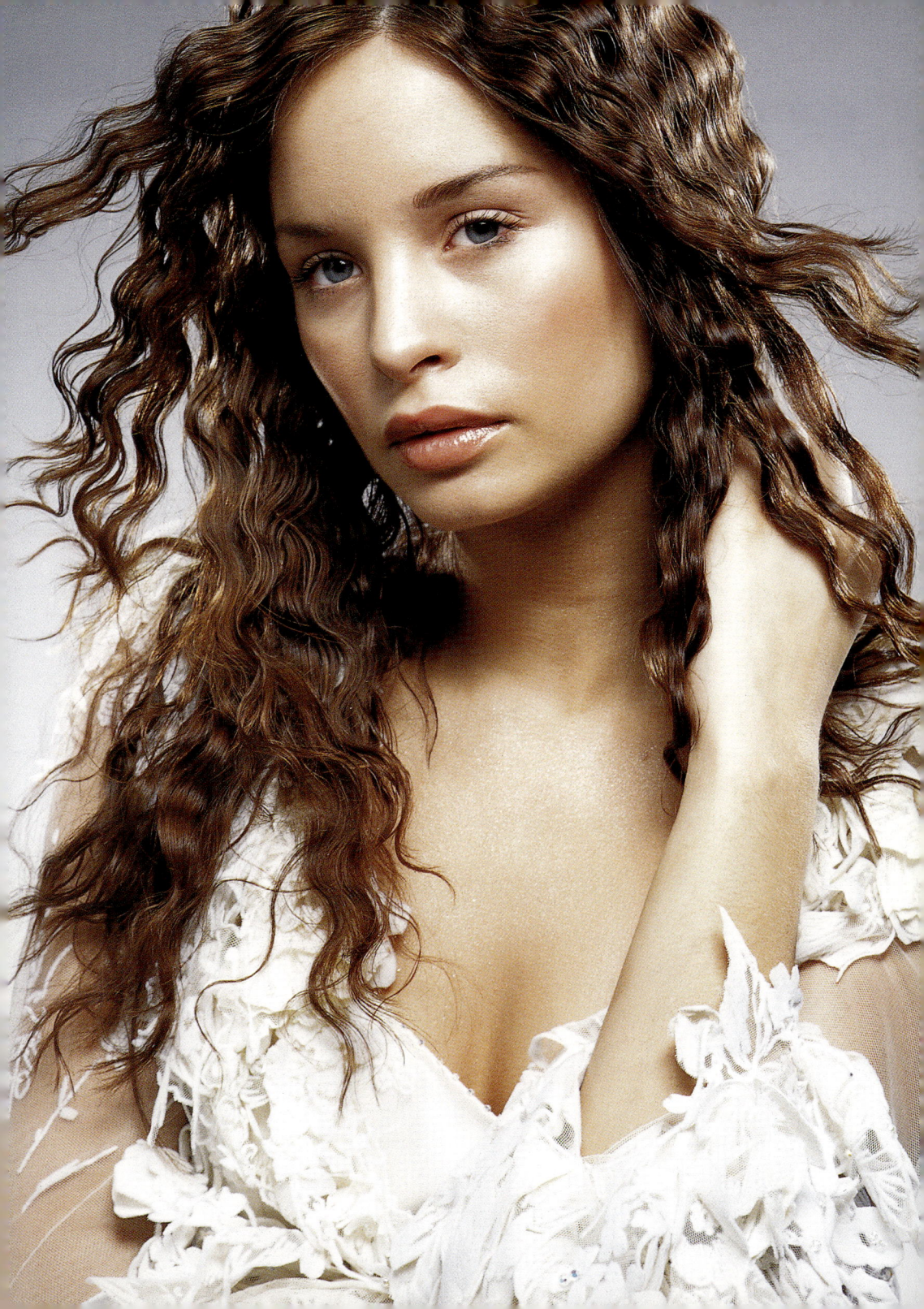

# country

The girl who goes for the country style loves all things pretty and natural, and that includes her look. Her dress will be a simple, feminine home-made affair; she'll carry a bouquet of wild flowers and wear a garland in her hair.

## hair solutions

Keep your hair unstructured and, if it's long, flowing loose over your shoulders. Flowers are the obvious choice for decoration, but keep them simple, small and dotted throughout the hair. Alternatively, take two sections of hair from the front and plait them, incorporating fine ribbons in shades of bright and baby pink; secure the back with a band and conceal it by wrapping a length of ribbon around it. A wild flower garland creates a feminine look for short hair.

**BELOW AND RIGHT**

The hair is sectioned into narrow segments, working forwards from the centre of the crown, twisted into tight knots and secured along the hairline with matt grips. The ends of the hair are left loose for a natural, romantic finish. For a dramatic look, decorate the knots with feathers that match your outfit.

**OVERLEAF**

Sections of the hair are sprayed using a fine-hold hairspray, and various sizes of tongs are used to create romantic ringlets. These can be left *au naturel* for a stronger look (left), or the curls can be broken up with fingers for a Lady Godiva look (right). Finish with gloss or serum to add curl definition. Various accessories can be used – from natural blooms to tiaras and strands of diamanté beads.

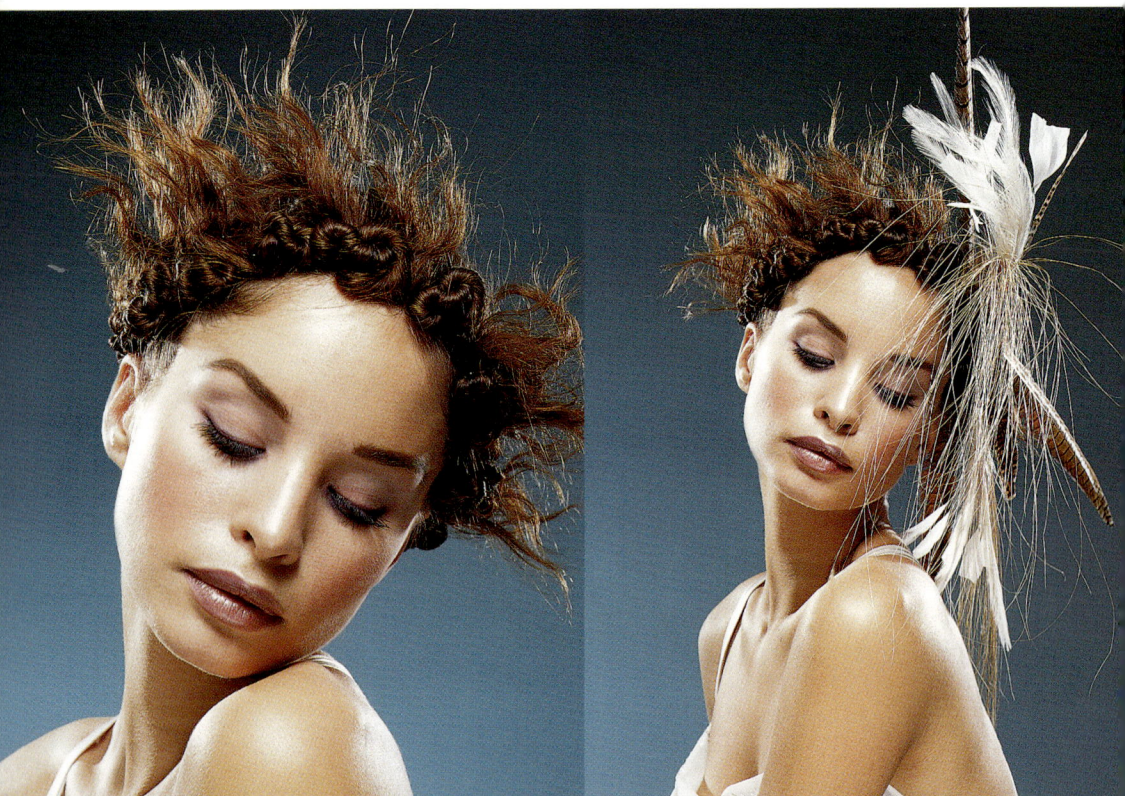

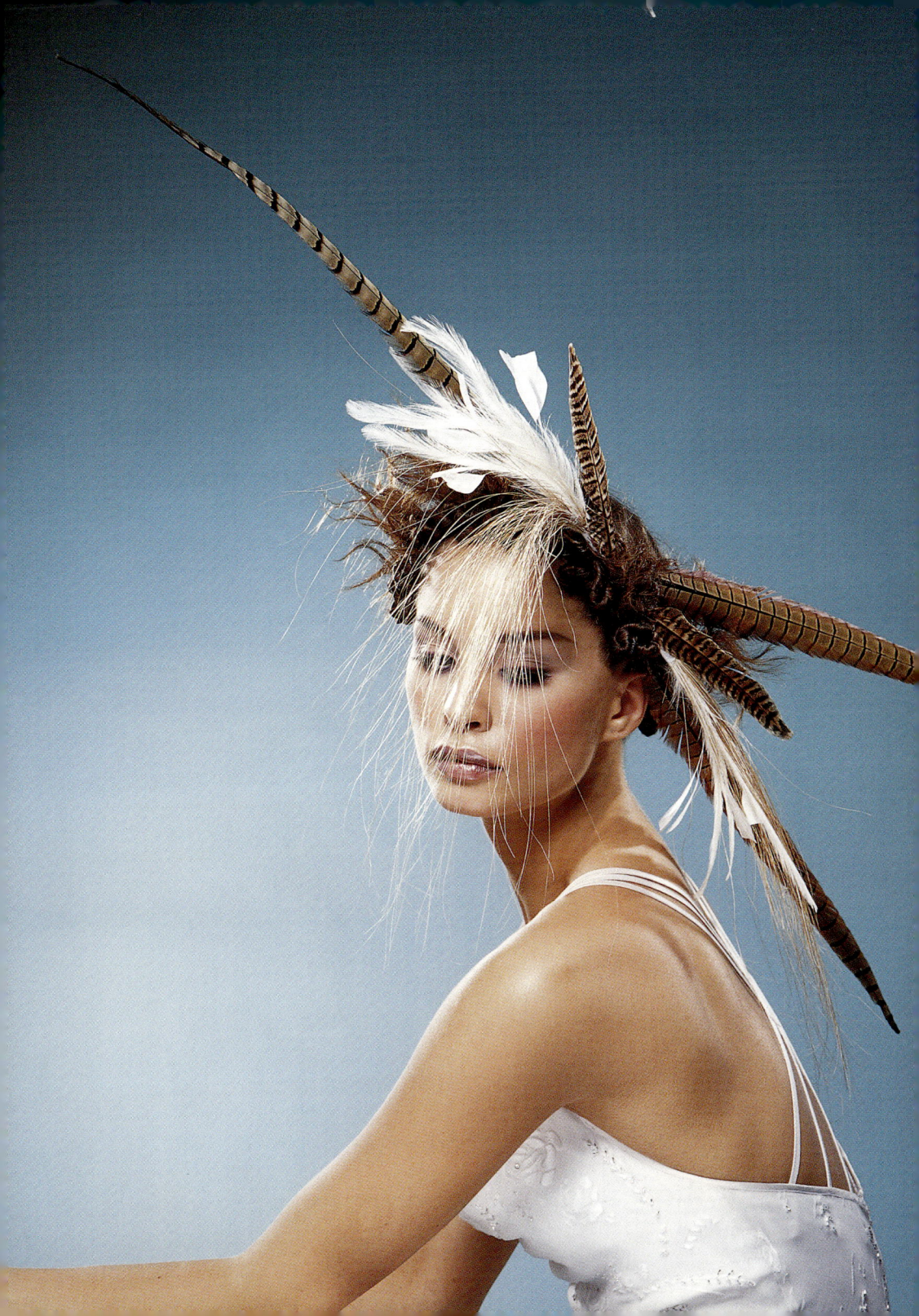

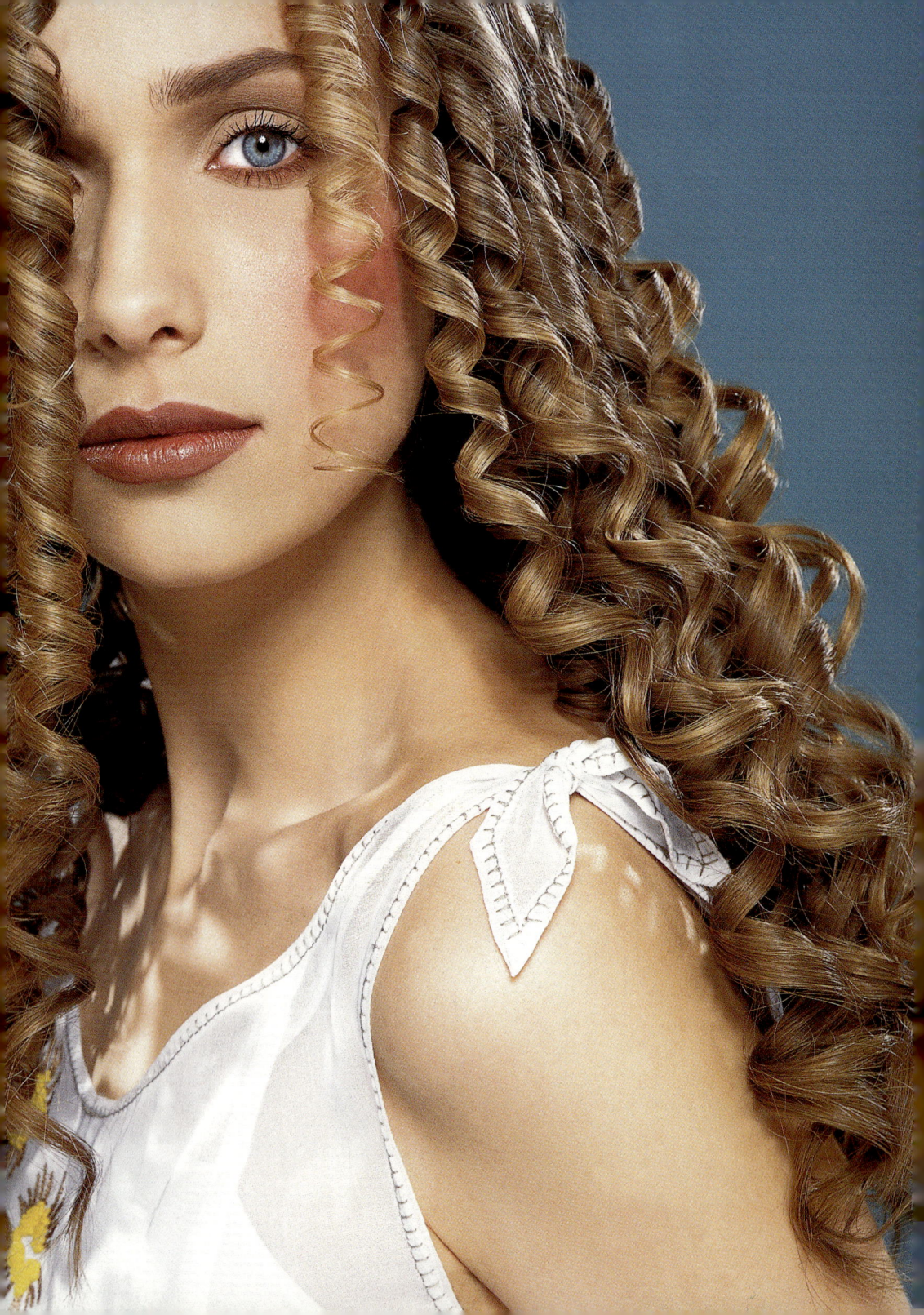

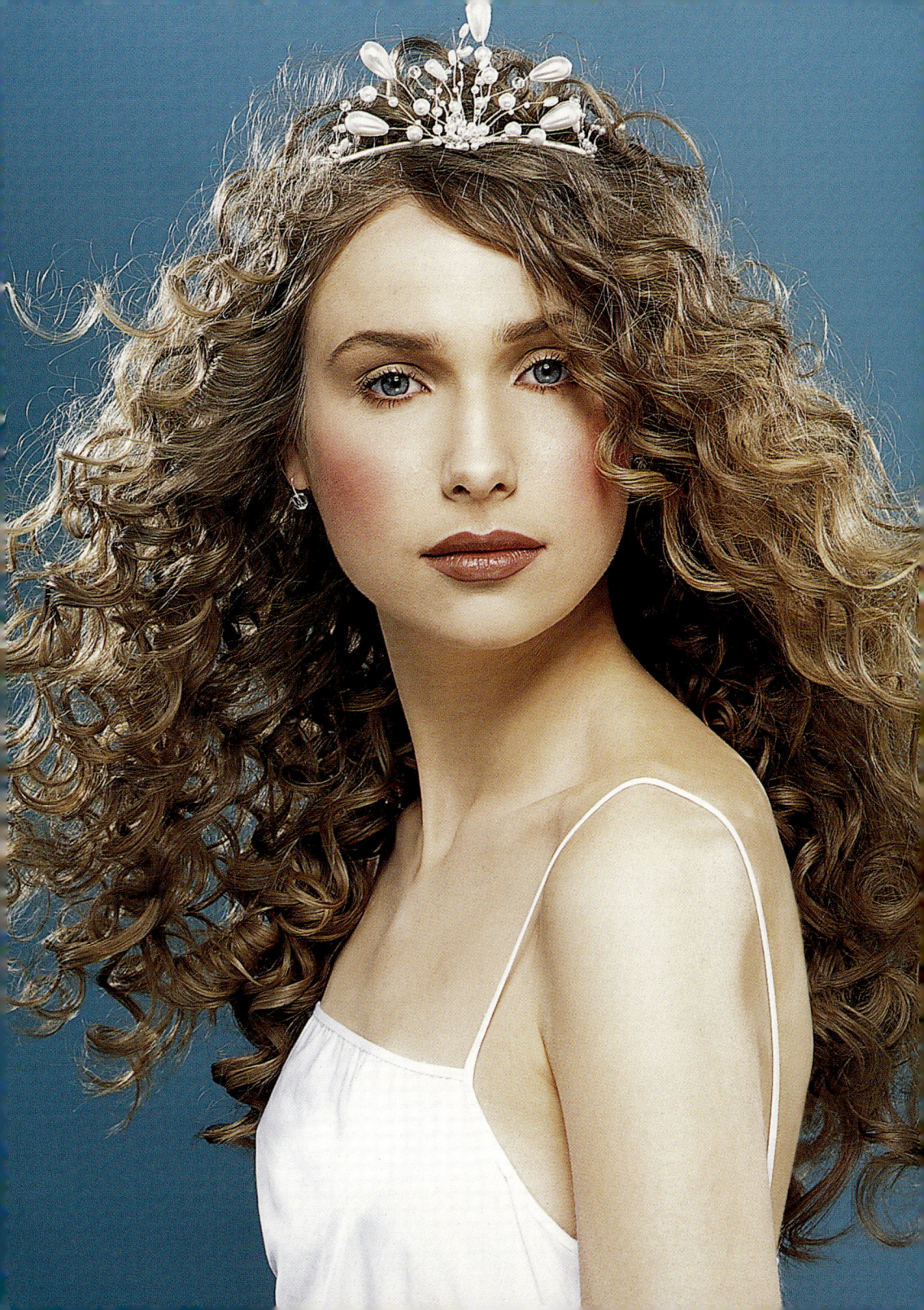

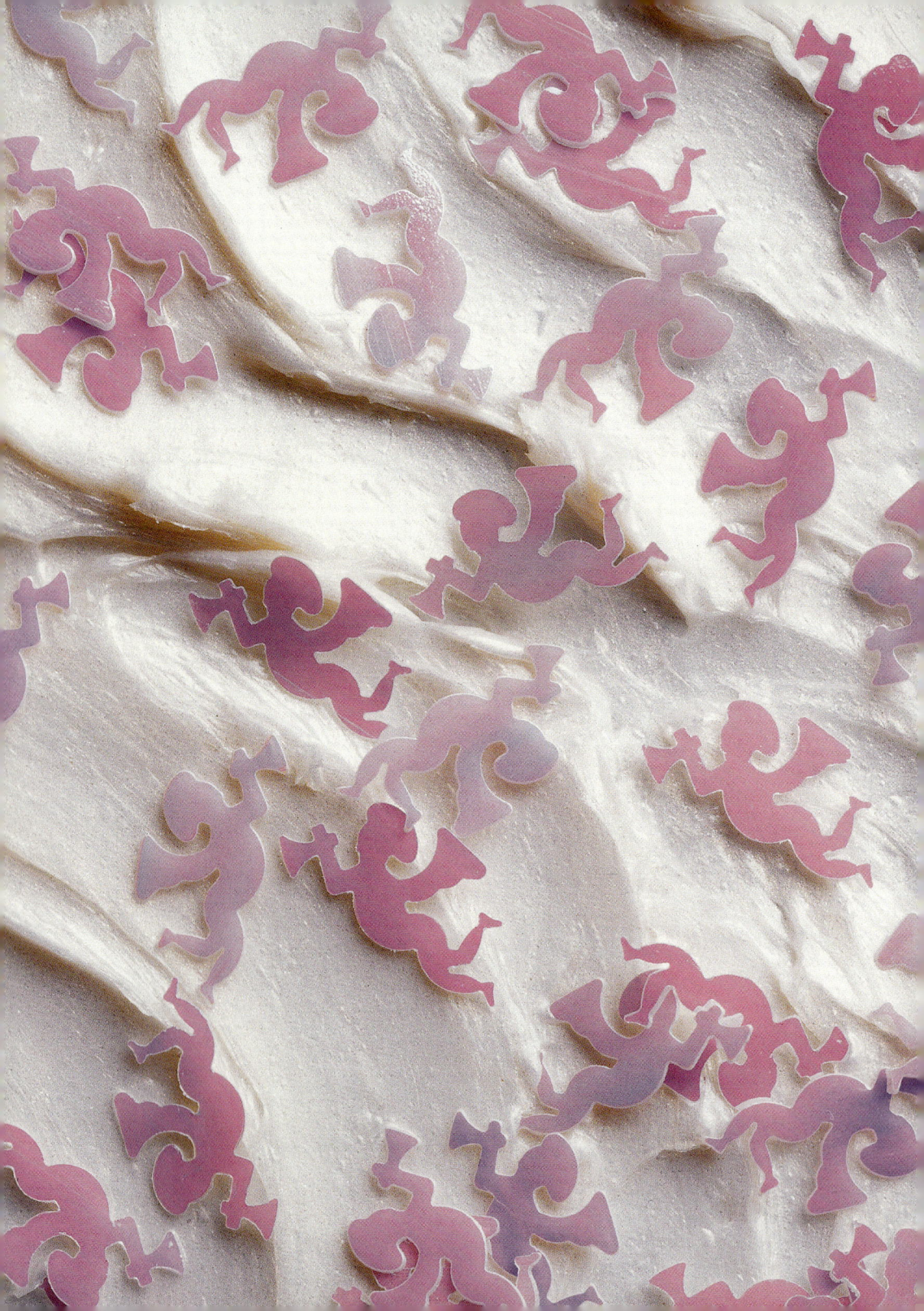

'**Grown up?**' exclaims Jaz's stylist, Zoe. She's been doing Jaz's hair since she was a junior stylist and has tried out all of her most directional looks on her. Jaz nods firmly. Her job at Astrid PR is everything she had hoped it would be, but she's started to think that she's being overlooked for promotion. Her cutting-edge look is great when she's dealing with designers or at the shows, but when it comes to important meetings she's often left behind. Is it because Astrid feels she can't deal with the business side of things? Or just that she can't get them to take her seriously in her present incarnation? Either way, she's ready for a change.

'I want to go for a classic, straight bob with a blunt fringe (bangs),' says Jaz. Zoe raises an eyebrow. 'Aha, the power bob. Trouble at work?' she asks. 'First of all, Jaz, you need to look like you, and that is so not your style. Secondly, it will drown your face. just look

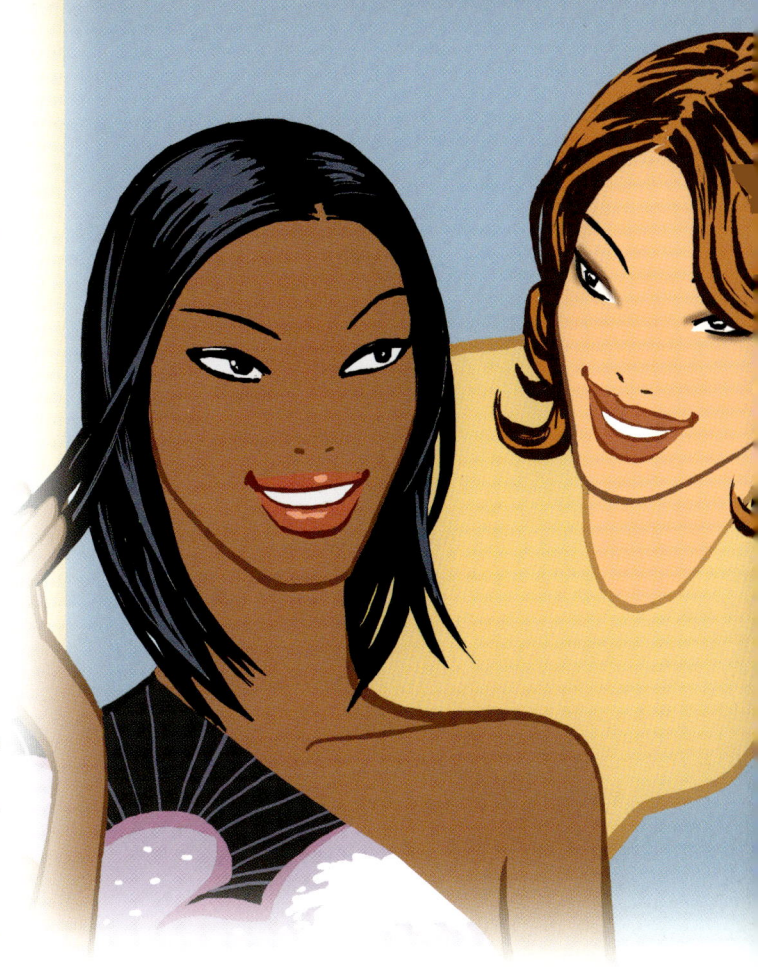

## ... jaz goes for a grown-up look

at your face shape.' Zoe is right; Jaz's slim heart-shaped face couldn't carry off such a look. 'Why don't we meet halfway?' Zoe suggests, 'and dye it back to its natural black, then cut it into a long bob, sloping down at the front and without a fringe. If we razor the ends, you can stop it from hanging in a single, heavy chunk. That way you have lots of versatility when you're not being Mrs Business Woman.'

'Sounds like you and I are changing places,' giggles Kate, slipping into the chair next to Jaz.
'Kate! What are you doing here?' asks Jaz, slightly unnerved to be caught dicing with conformity.
'I'm getting back to my roots, literally,' says Kate. 'My highlights from the holiday are growing out, so I'm having a vegetable colour put on to bring back my normal titian colour.' Jaz eyes her old school friend in the mirror. She looks great; she hasn't used her hair straighteners since her return, letting her natural curl reassert itself with a vengeance. She seems so much more confident and relaxed than the girl who went away.
'Is there something you're not telling me?' Jaz enquires. Kate smiles as Zoe leads Jaz away to wash her hair.
'No,' she says. 'It's just that some things are better left unspoilt.'

GET THE LOOK 39

# urbanite

GET THE LOOK

Everything in her life is luxurious but with a thoroughly modern edge. She's a high-maintenance girl whose wardrobe is filled with elegant, well-cut clothes and whose look is one of understated glamour. Naturally, her wedding outfit is no exception. She'll be wearing an exquisitely cut white trouser suit with a plunging neckline revealing a fair amount of bare *décolletage*. Jewellery will be simple and modern, and a flower-ball bouquet will be dangling from her slender wrist.

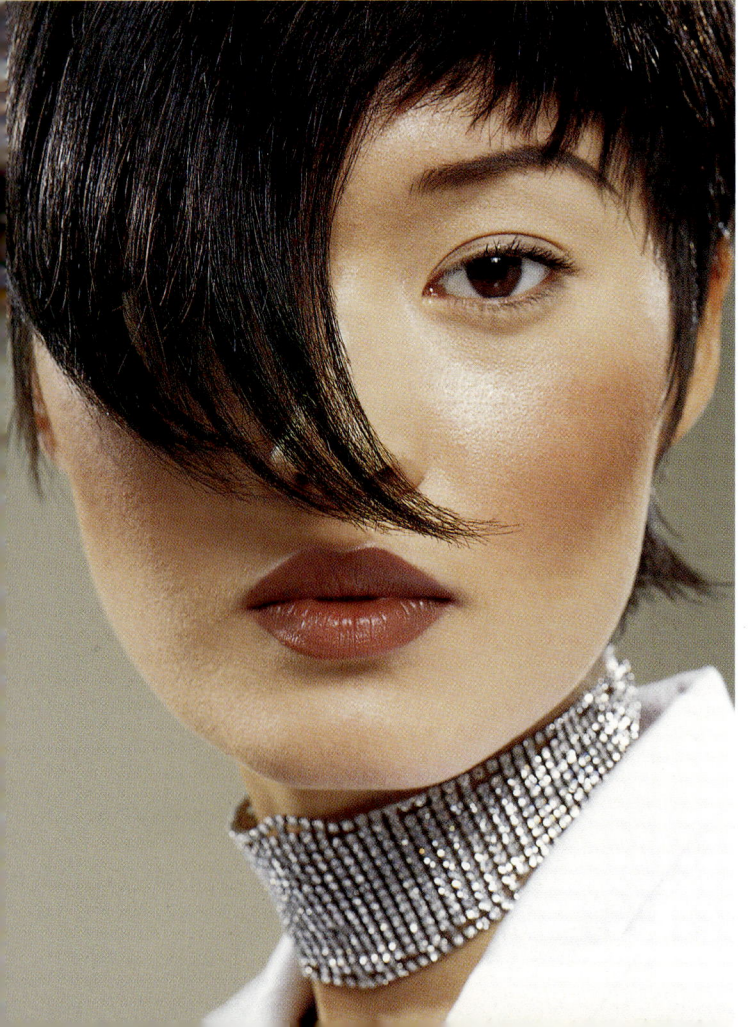

## hair solutions

Short hair naturally complements this sharp look, while mid-length hair is best in a 1920s-style bob. Long hair is great poker-straight with an extreme side parting and a section pulled back into a feather headdress. Keep it simple, with the accent on impeccable condition.

### LEFT AND RIGHT

For the textured look (right), the hair is tousled using wet-look gel to give a glossy, almost glass-like finish. The hair on the crown is styled using the fingers to give texture, height and a spiky finish. If you have short hair but want a longer look, use a ¾ hairpiece to add length and interest around the face (left).

### OVERLEAF LEFT

The hair is scrunch-dried using a blow-dry primer spray for volume and texture. It is swept back into a high ponytail, and backbrushed and sculpted into the required shape. The style is finished with a firm-hold hairspray and a necklace or bracelet pinned to the front of the 'sculpture'. A veil-type fringe is also an option.

### OVERLEAF RIGHT

The hair is slicked back into a mid-height ponytail and set on heated rollers. The curls are broken up with the fingers and piled into a clear, natural hairnet, secured with fine pins. A feathered comb can be added to the side of the bun.

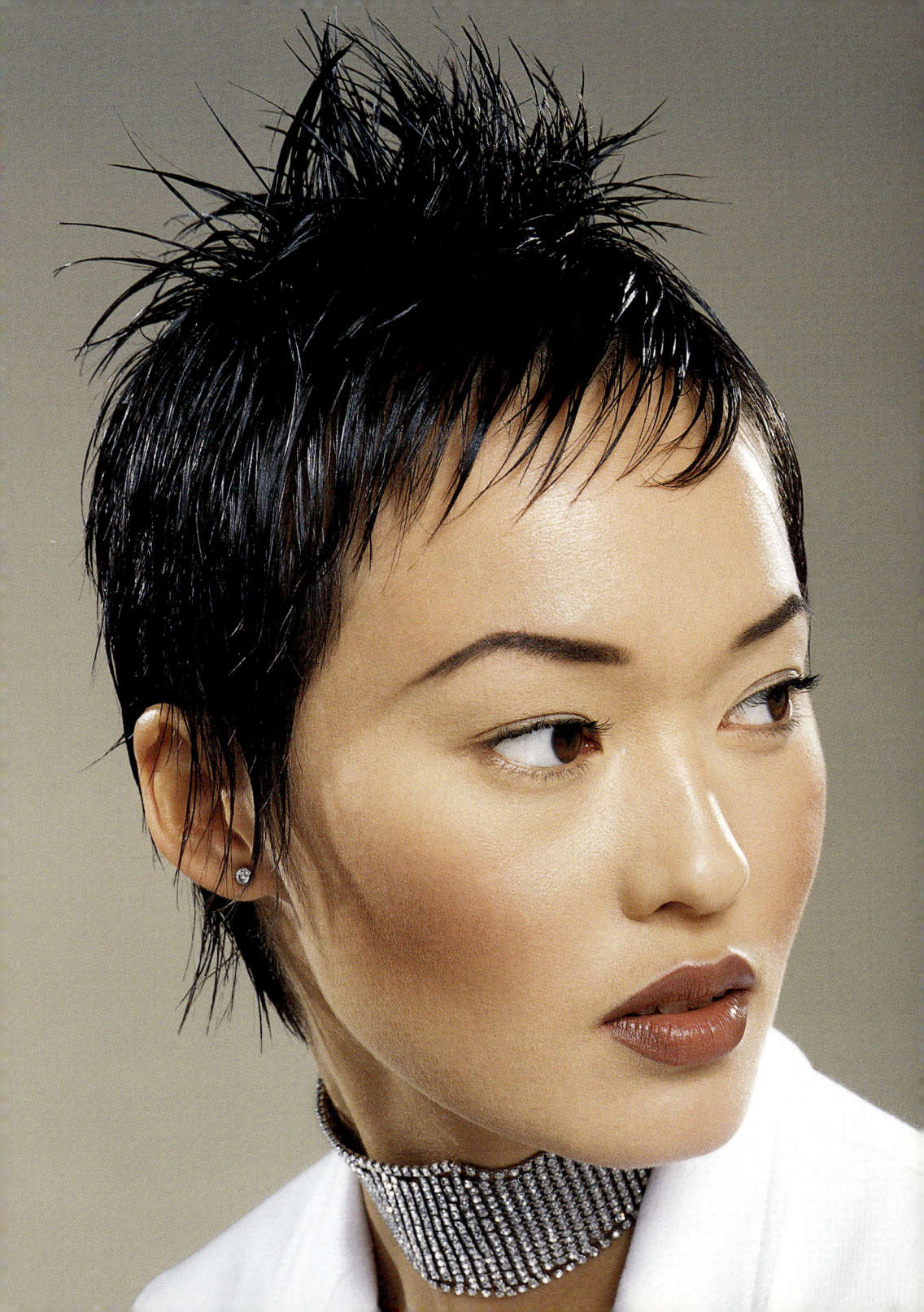

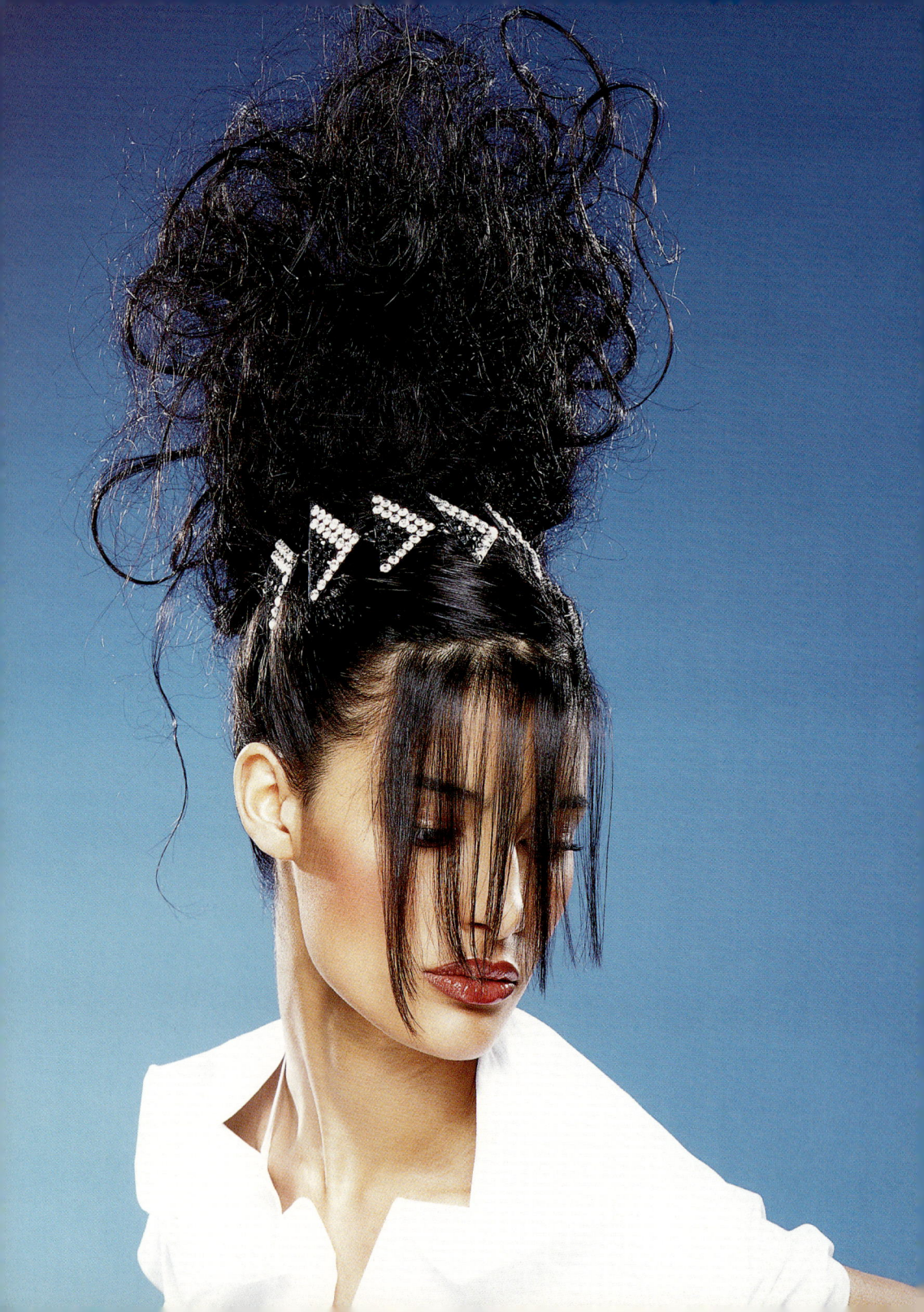

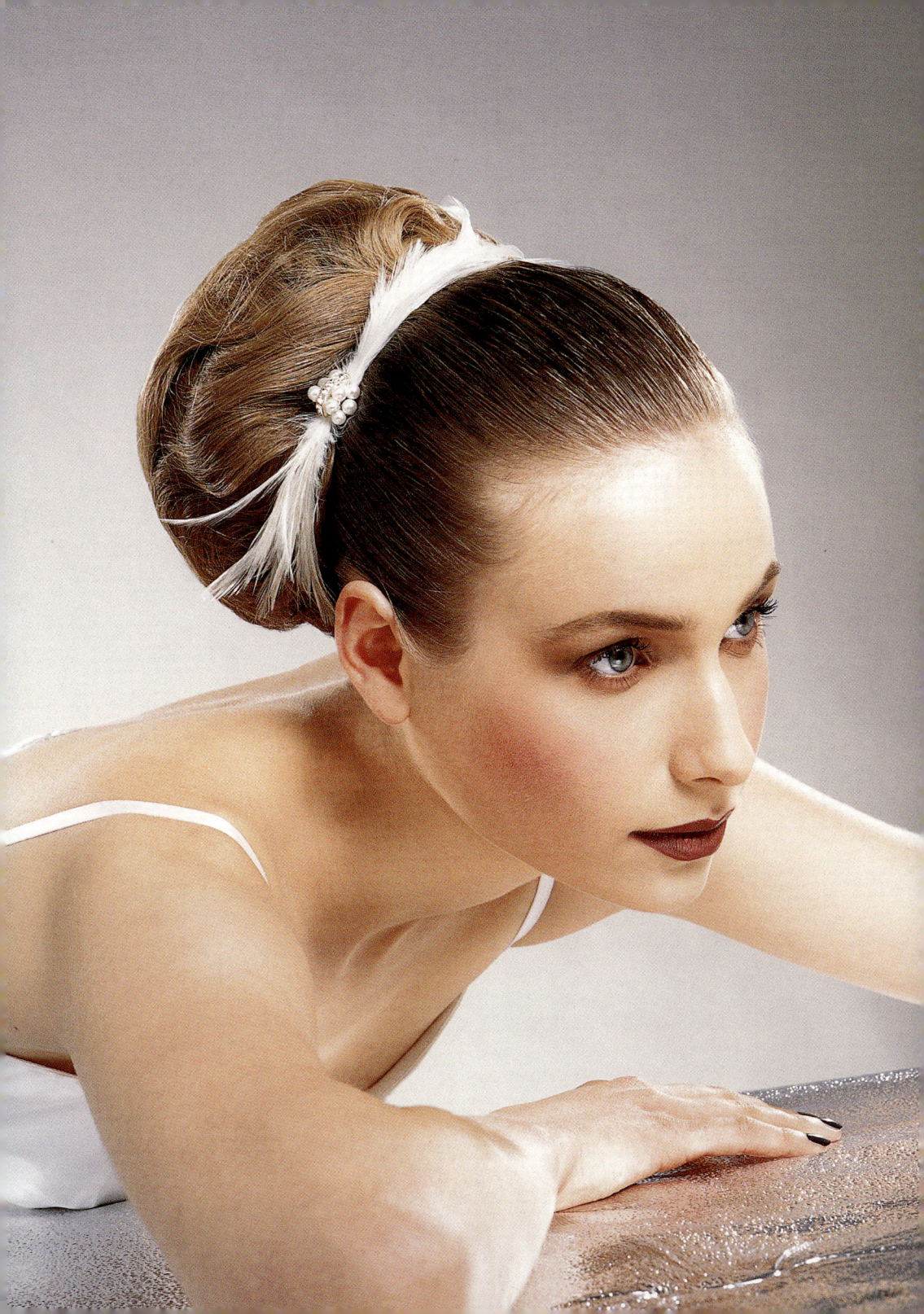

# audrey

Her biggest style influence is, of course, Audrey Hepburn in *Breakfast at Tiffany's*. She always looks well groomed and classically elegant – her uniform is crisp linen shift dresses for summer and neat pencil skirts and fitted sweaters for winter. For her wedding, she'll be wearing a sleeveless column dress in off-white satin, and carrying either a tight posy of cream roses tied with pale blue ribbon or a single long-stemmed amaryllis or lily.

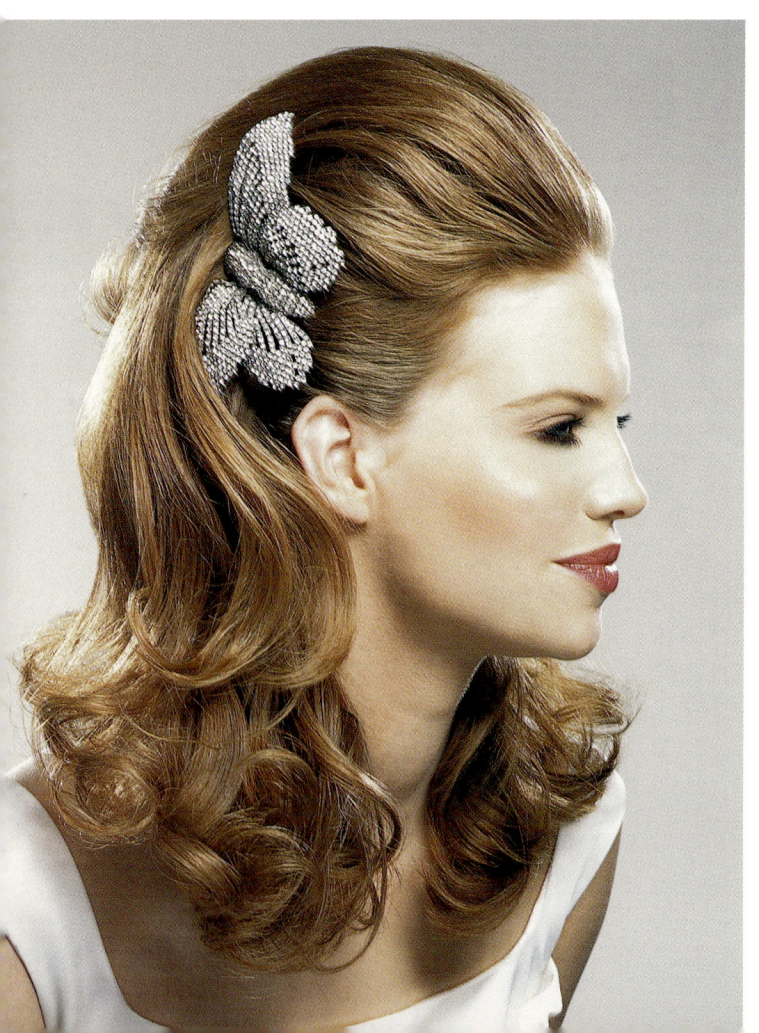

## hair solutions

Smoothing your long hair into a neat chignon, with a subtle tiara and a satin-trimmed shoulder-length veil, is a perfectly classic look. Mid-length hair looks great accessorized with an Alice band and mini-veil, while vivid orchids and green tendrils secured behind one ear are ideal for short hair.

**LEFT**

The hair is set on medium-sized rollers using a fine flexi-hold hairspray and allowed to cool totally before gently removing them. The curls are broken up using a large-toothed comb and the root area of the crown is backcombed. The sides are smoothed back and pinned with matt grips. A decorative comb completes the look.

**RIGHT**

The hair is swept up into a neat high ponytail in the centre of the head. It is then set on heated rollers, which are removed when they are totally cool. The hair is pulled through two bun rings over which the curls are placed and pinned. A necklace can be pinned across the hairline for decoration.

### HAIR SNIP

BALANCE IS ABSOLUTELY ESSENTIAL. DO NOT GO TOO BIG IF YOU ARE TALL, BUT TRY BIGGER HAIR IF YOU ARE ON THE SHORT SIDE – YOU NEVER KNOW, YOU MAY LOVE IT.

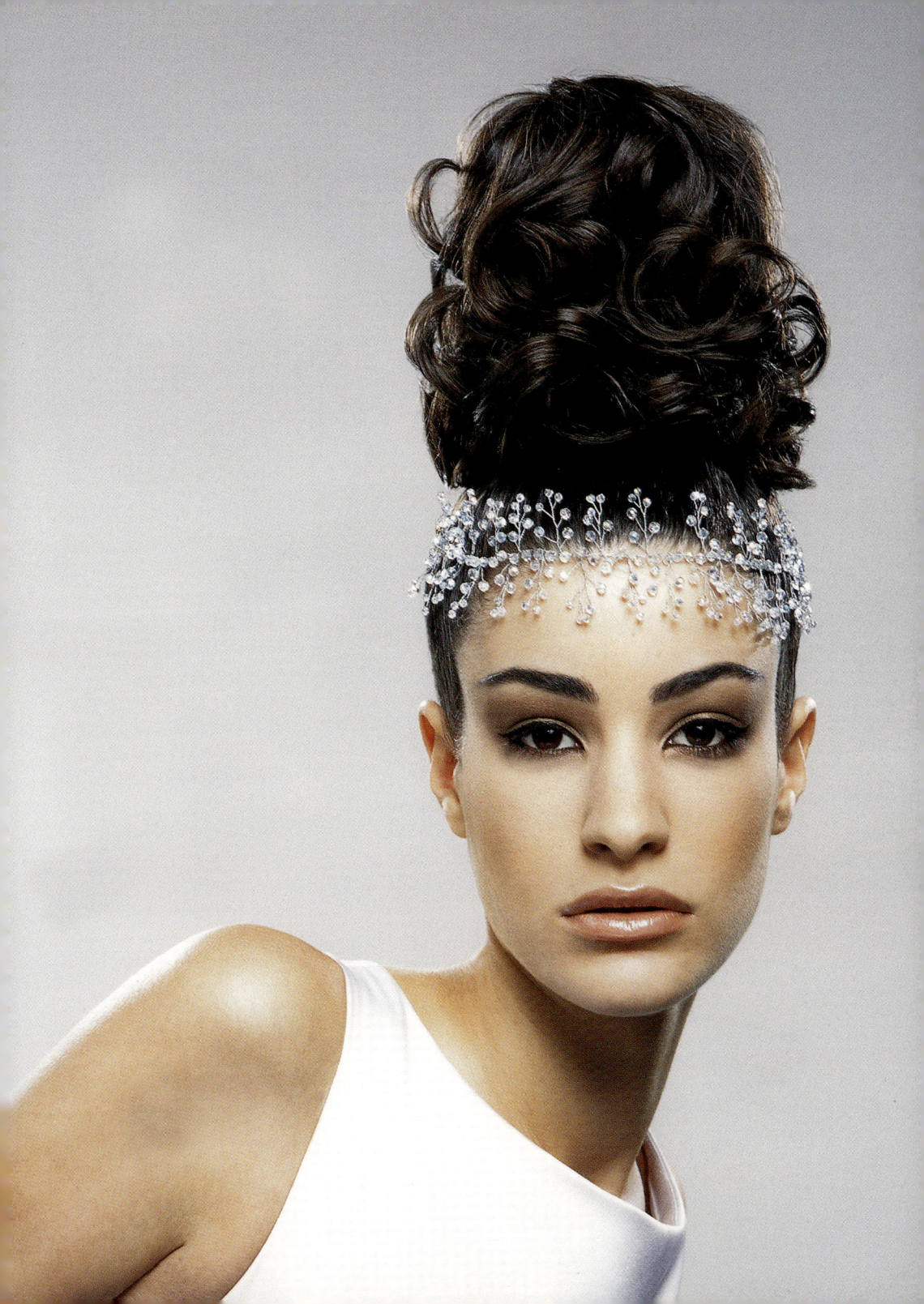

# classic

'Refined good taste' are this girl's watchwords. She always looks immaculate, even on casual days. For work she wears beautifully tailored suits and relaxes at the weekend in smart but fashionable denim or cords. She thrives on tradition and ceremony, and never more so than at her own wedding. Her elegant empire-line gown in duchesse satin is offset with a frothy white veil and a trailing bouquet of white flowers and green foliage for a timelessly stylish look.

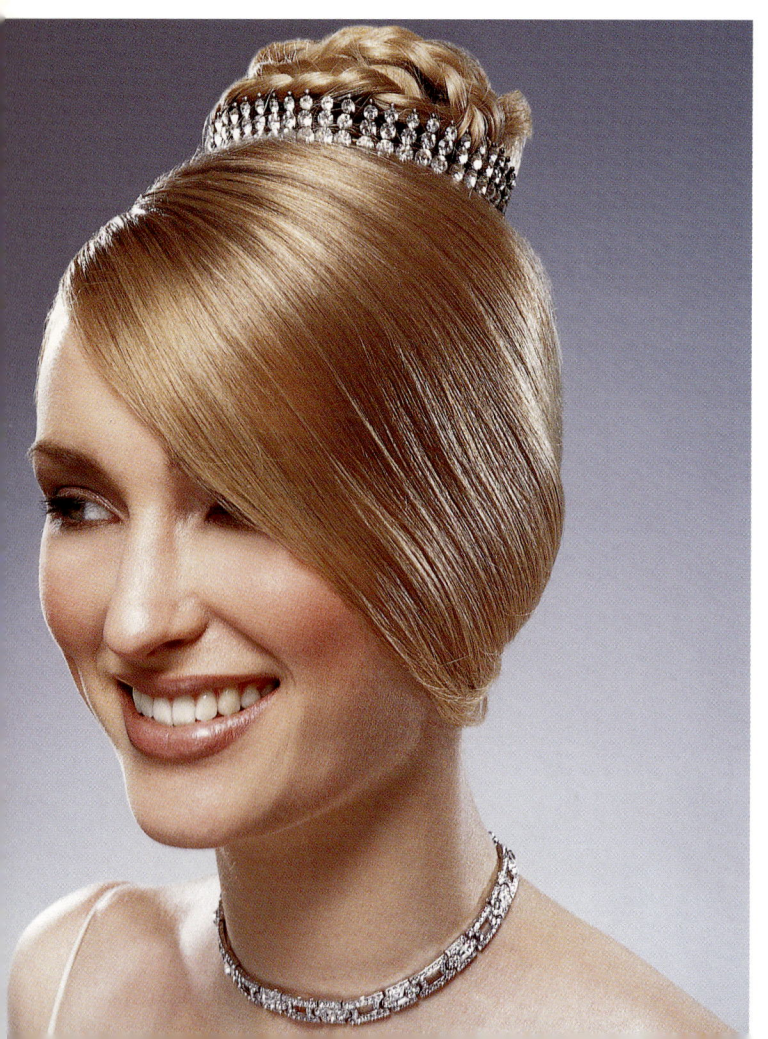

## hair solutions

This is perfect for those who want the quintessential bridal look of veil and tiara. A crown tiara is great on short hair, while long hair demands to be piled up high. For fine or mid-length hair, try adding a hairpiece.

### LEFT AND RIGHT
Ultra-glossy hair is swept back and secured into a French pleat using fine pins and matt grips. A small circular tiara is placed onto the crown, and a plaited section of hair is positioned inside and held in place with hair pins and hairspray.

### OVERLEAF LEFT
The root area of freshly blow-dried or set hair is backbrushed. The nape section is swept up to the crown and secured with matt grips. The top section is brought over, wound down onto the mid-section and fastened with matt grips to create a soft roll. Accessories or feathers can be added to the base of the roll.

### OVERLEAF RIGHT
The hair is set on medium-sized rollers using a fine flexi-hold hairspray. When cool, the rollers are removed and the curls are broken up using a large-toothed comb. Using fingers as a comb, the hair is shaped around the face in large sweeping waves. For gentle hold, hairspray is applied to the fingers and run through the hair.

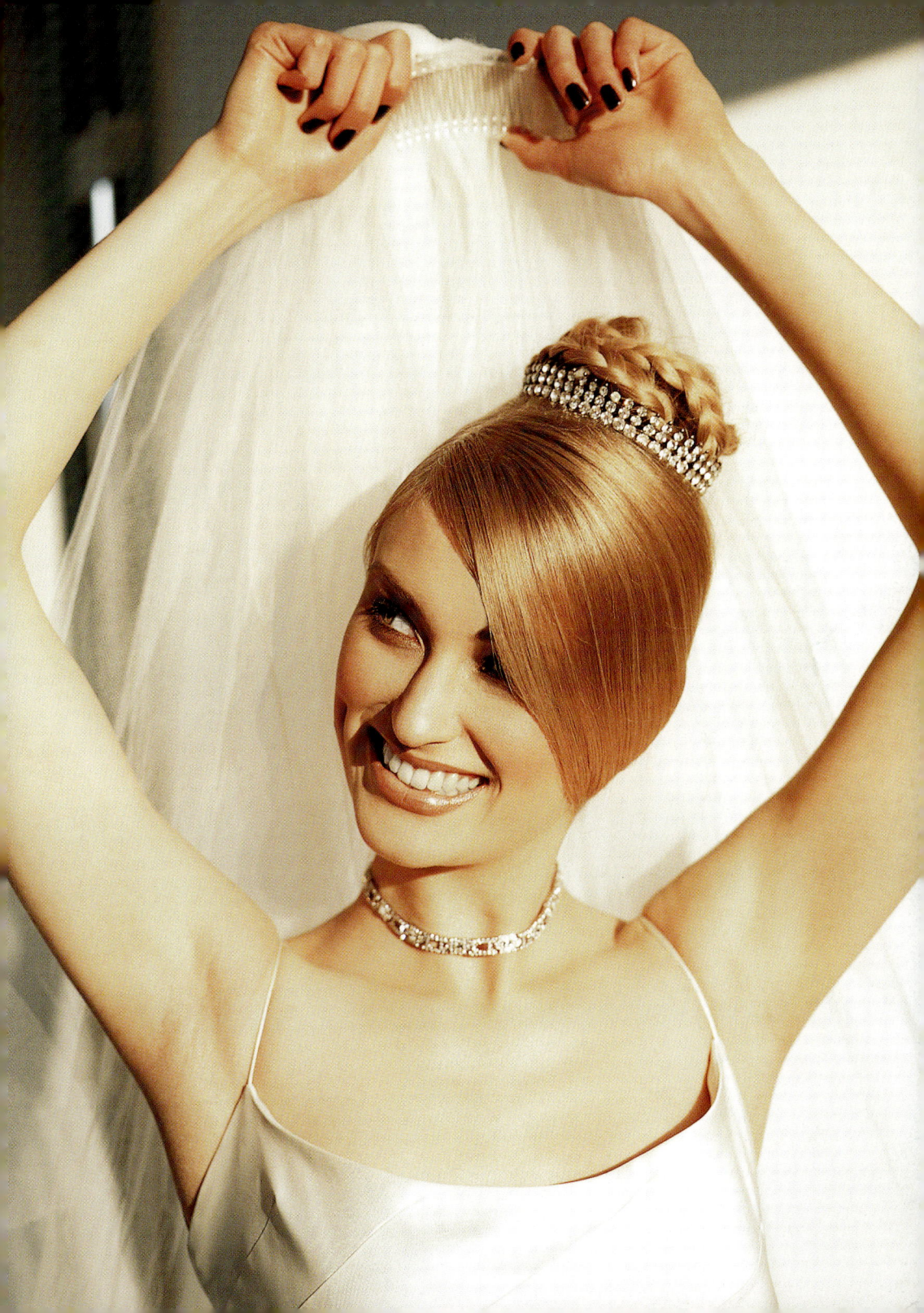

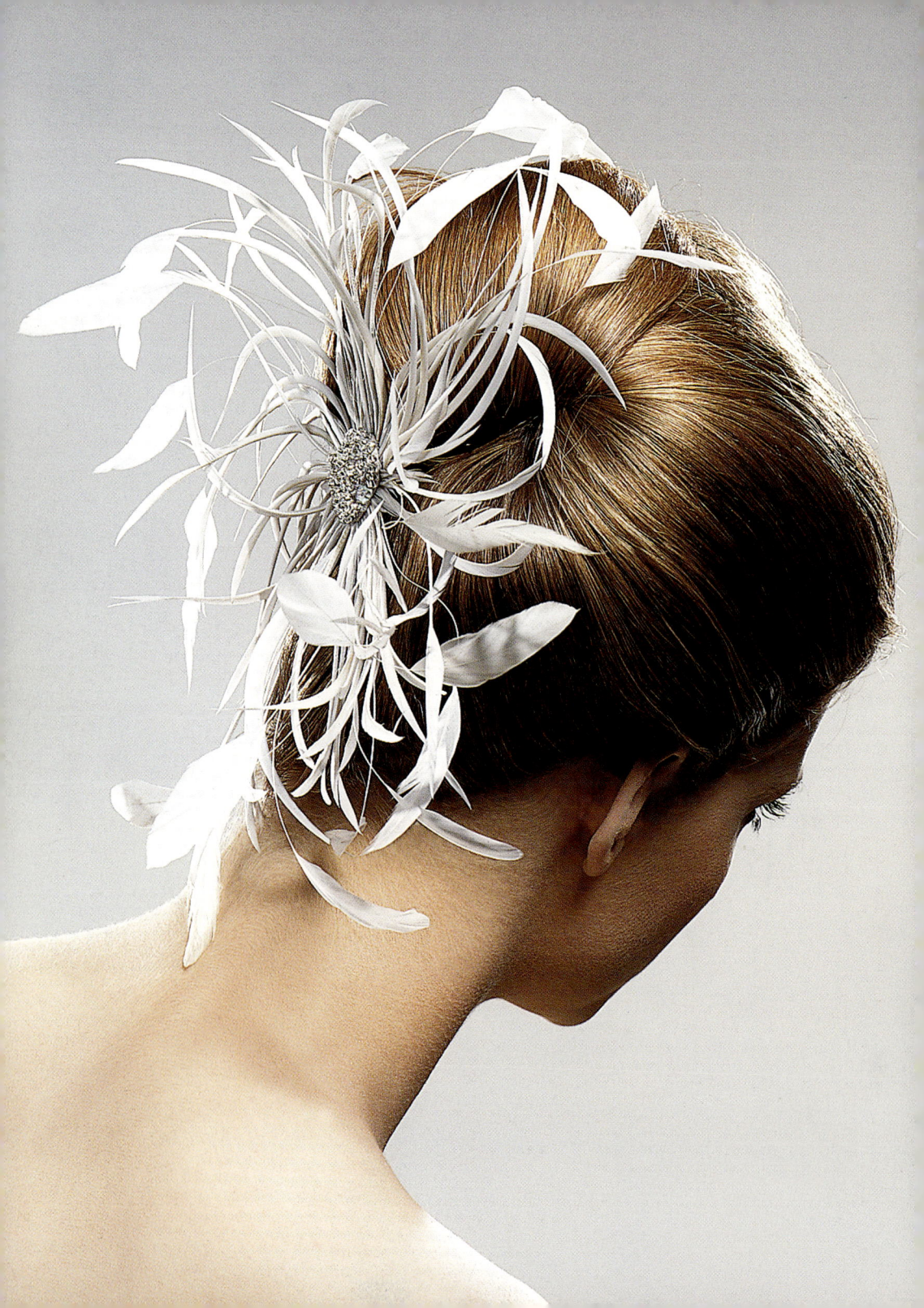

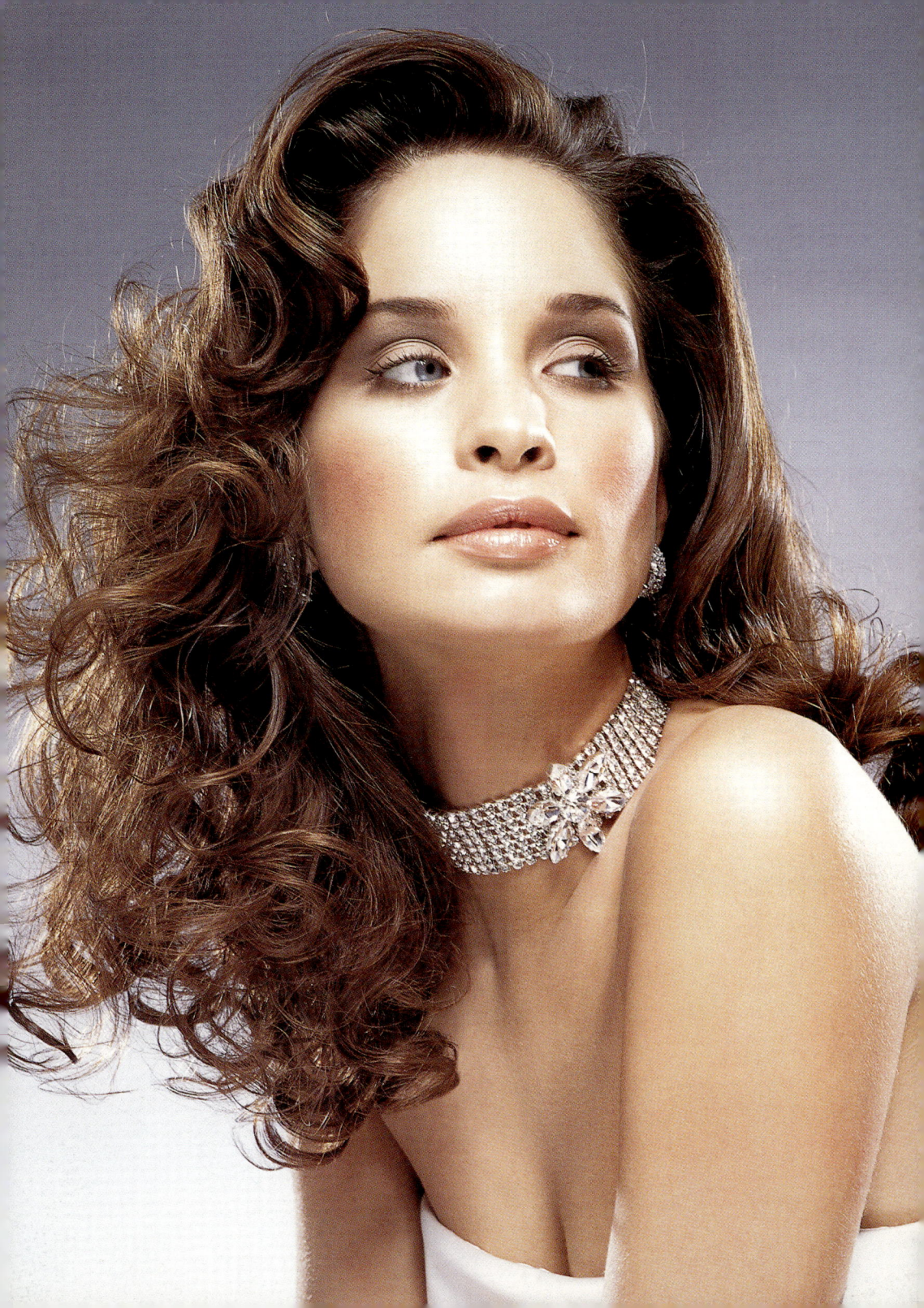

# rock chick

This girl loves to play – and her wedding day will be no exception. Her usual uniform is skin-tight denim, tiny ripped T-shirts, leather cuffs and high-heeled snake-skin ankle boots. Her bridal version will comprise a very short skirt, a slash-neck top and fishnets – all in snowy white. She won't carry flowers, but will finish off the look with a diamanté collar and cuffs, smoky eyes and hair with serious attitude.

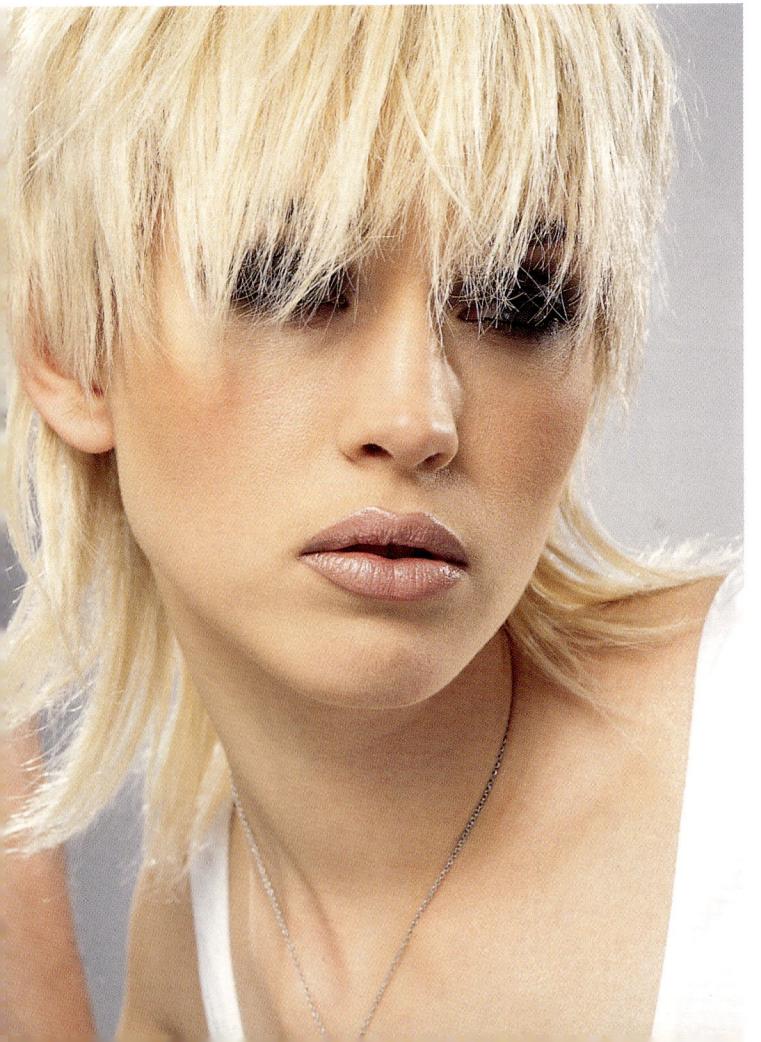

## hair solutions

Regardless of length, the look here is big, big, big. Lots of texture and backcombing will give long hair that sexy just-about-to-fall-into-bed-head look – but remember to use products only at the roots, or the hair will be weighed down. With shorter hair, try a tiara on a choppy, textured cut. On any length, don't forget height at the crown.

**LEFT AND RIGHT**
For a classic rock-chick look, the hair is dyed 'peroxide' blonde and cut dry using a razor to inject some attitude into this modern style. Wax is used to give a matt, chunky finish and a sparkling crystal tiara makes this look a little more feminine.

**OVERLEAF LEFT**
For an ultra-modern rock-chick look, the hair is cut randomly using texturizing scissors and coloured with a variety of red and petrol tones to create an edgy effect.

**OVERLEAF RIGHT**
The hair is blow-dried using blow-dry priming spray to give volume and create a tendril effect. It is then pulled up into ponytails along the centre of the head in a mohican formation, then randomly placed and pinned to give a soft but edgy finish. Fake hairpieces can be added for extra drama if desired.

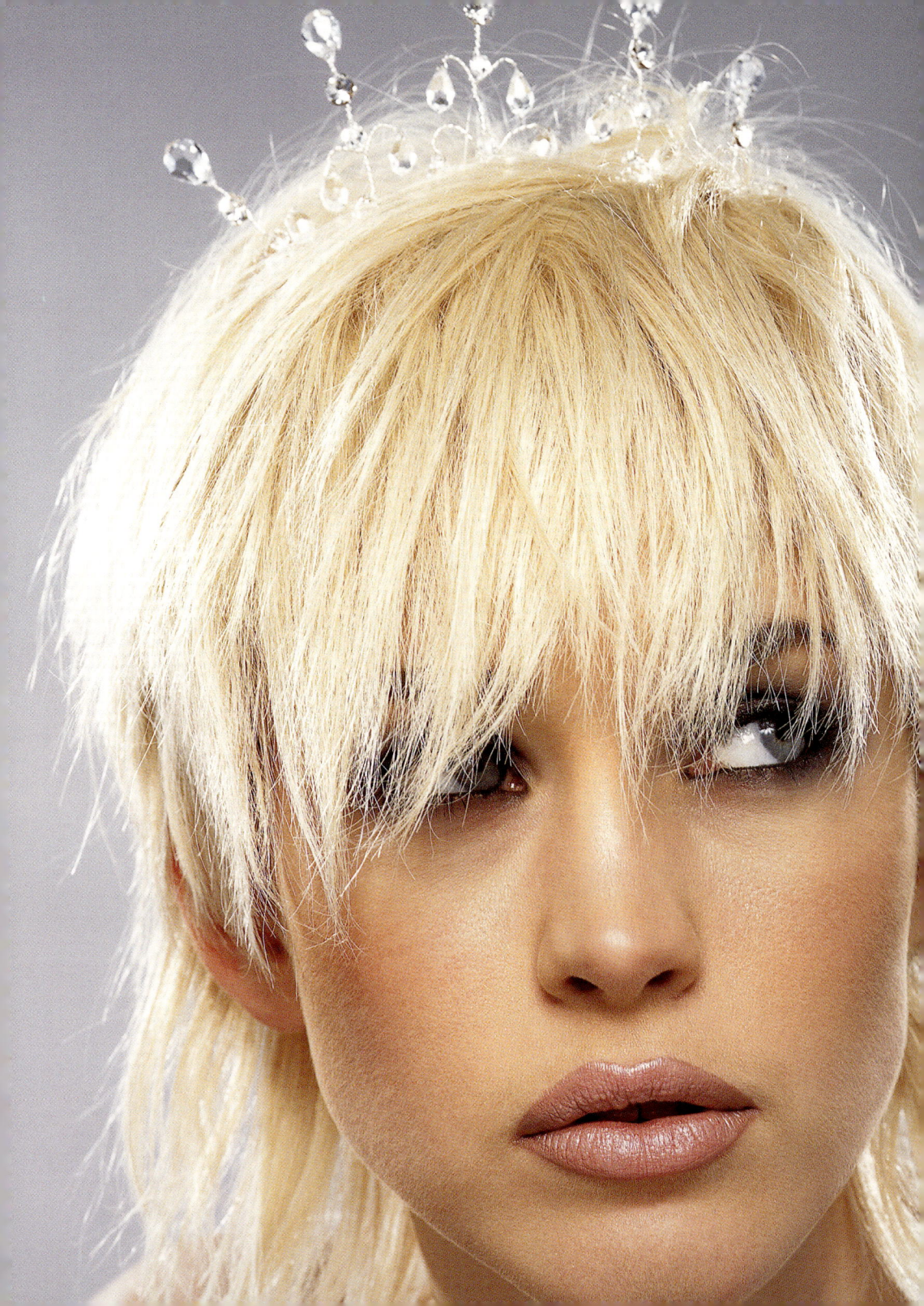

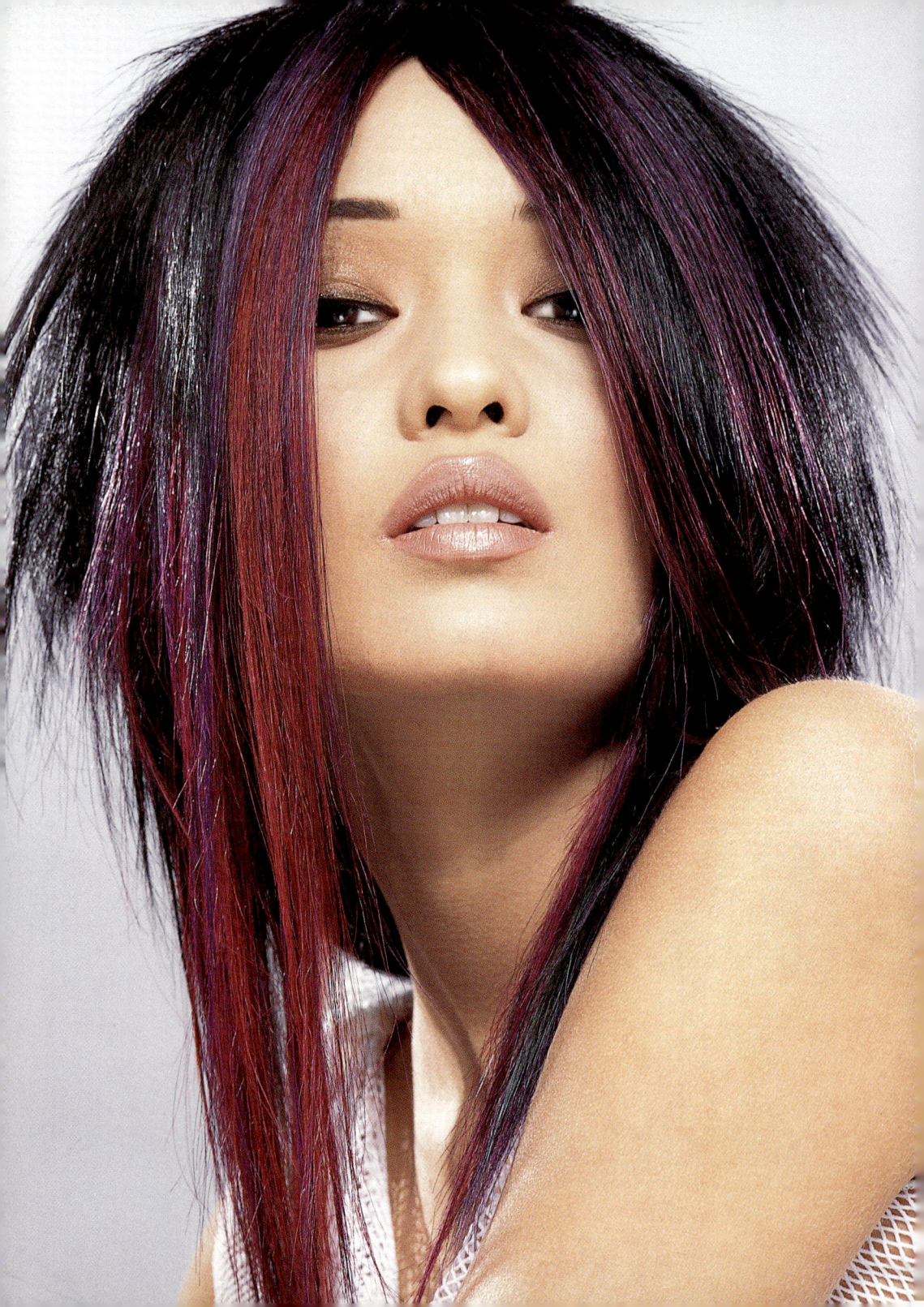

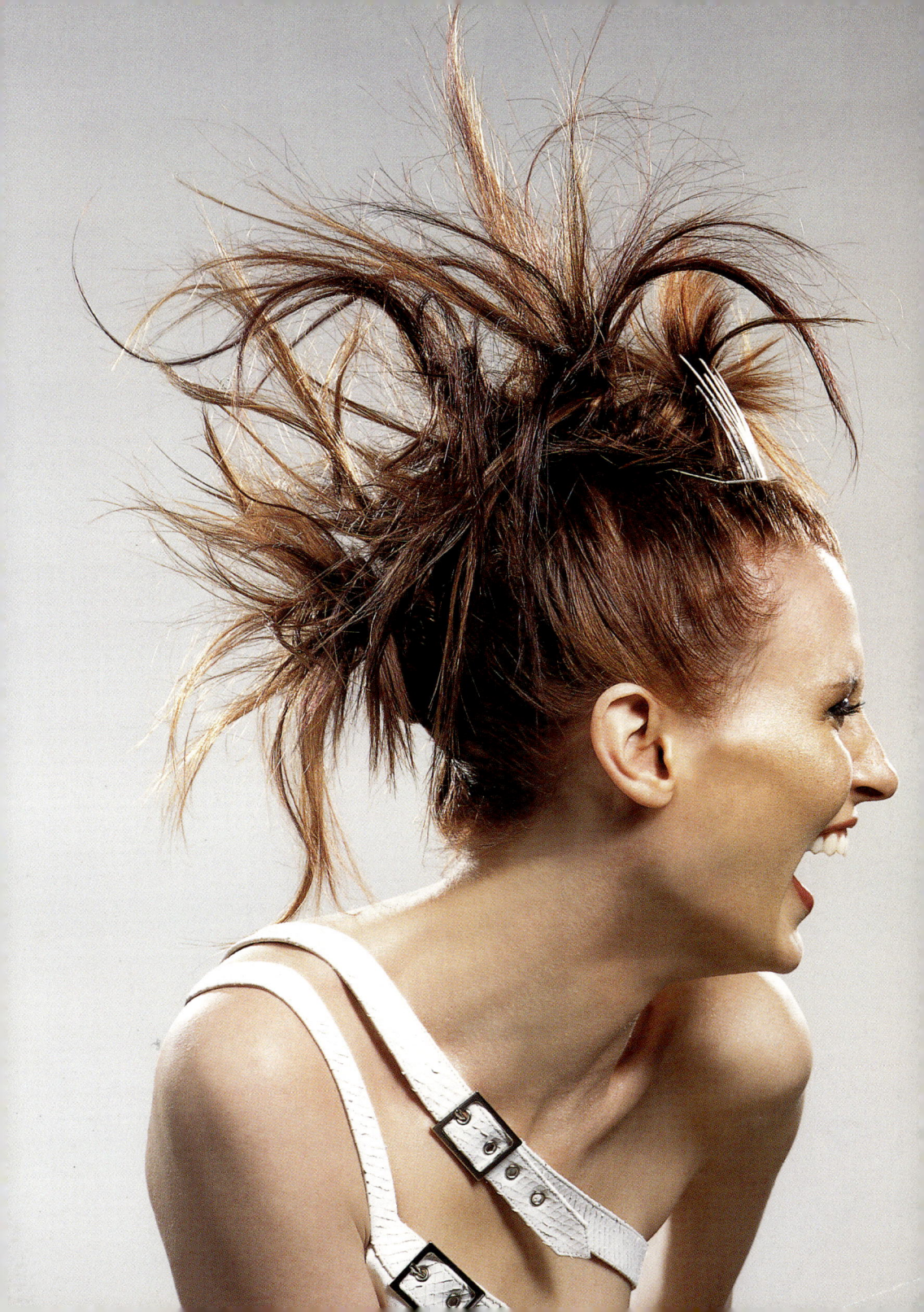

# fashionista

Luckily, marriage is back in fashion and this bride-to-be has embraced it with as much enthusiasm as she always has for designer sales. Her dress will be *couture*, of course – a bright pink slip covered with transparent, spider-web lace. She'll be sashaying down the aisle as though it were a catwalk, wearing perilously high strappy slingbacks. Flowers are a wrist corsage or choker, consisting of a single orchid.

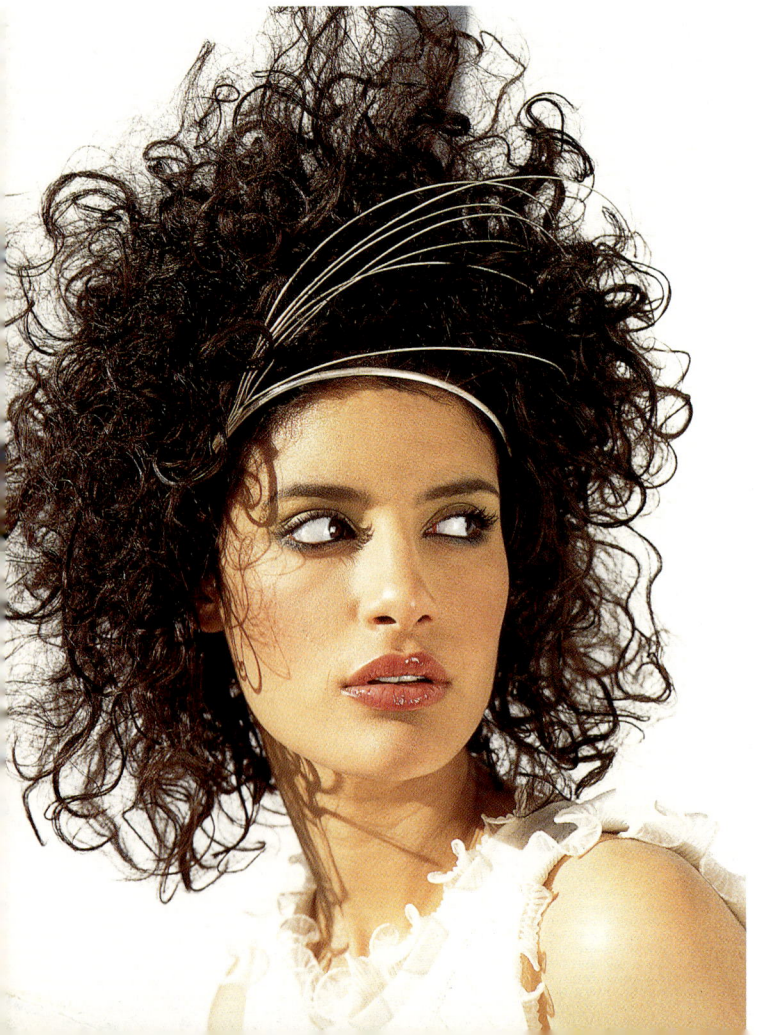

## hair solutions

Whatever the length of your hair, its condition is vital, so make sure you book in for some conditioning treatments well before the big day. On long hair, instead of a traditional tiara, try pinning a necklace across the forehead over unstructured big hair. A shorter style can look stunning when the hair is textured and single diamanté studs are clipped into it. Medium-length hair looks feminine in a shaggy style – create the separation by twisting damp, moussed hair into bands and leaving it to dry. Beaded flower clips can be used to pull hair back and draw attention to the face.

**LEFT**
This is achieved with a 'scrumpling' technique, which provides a modern take on curly hair. The hair is drenched with mousse, scrumpled down and pinned, then left to dry. The pins are removed and the hair is formed and shaped into the required style. A firm-hold hairspray sets and holds the style. Add a modern band or tiara to maximize the dramatic impact.

**RIGHT**
The hair is swept back into a twist, leaving the ends to splay out to one side of the head in a fan effect. Wax is used to give definition and texture to the ends. A theatrical necklace works well as a modern skull-cap.

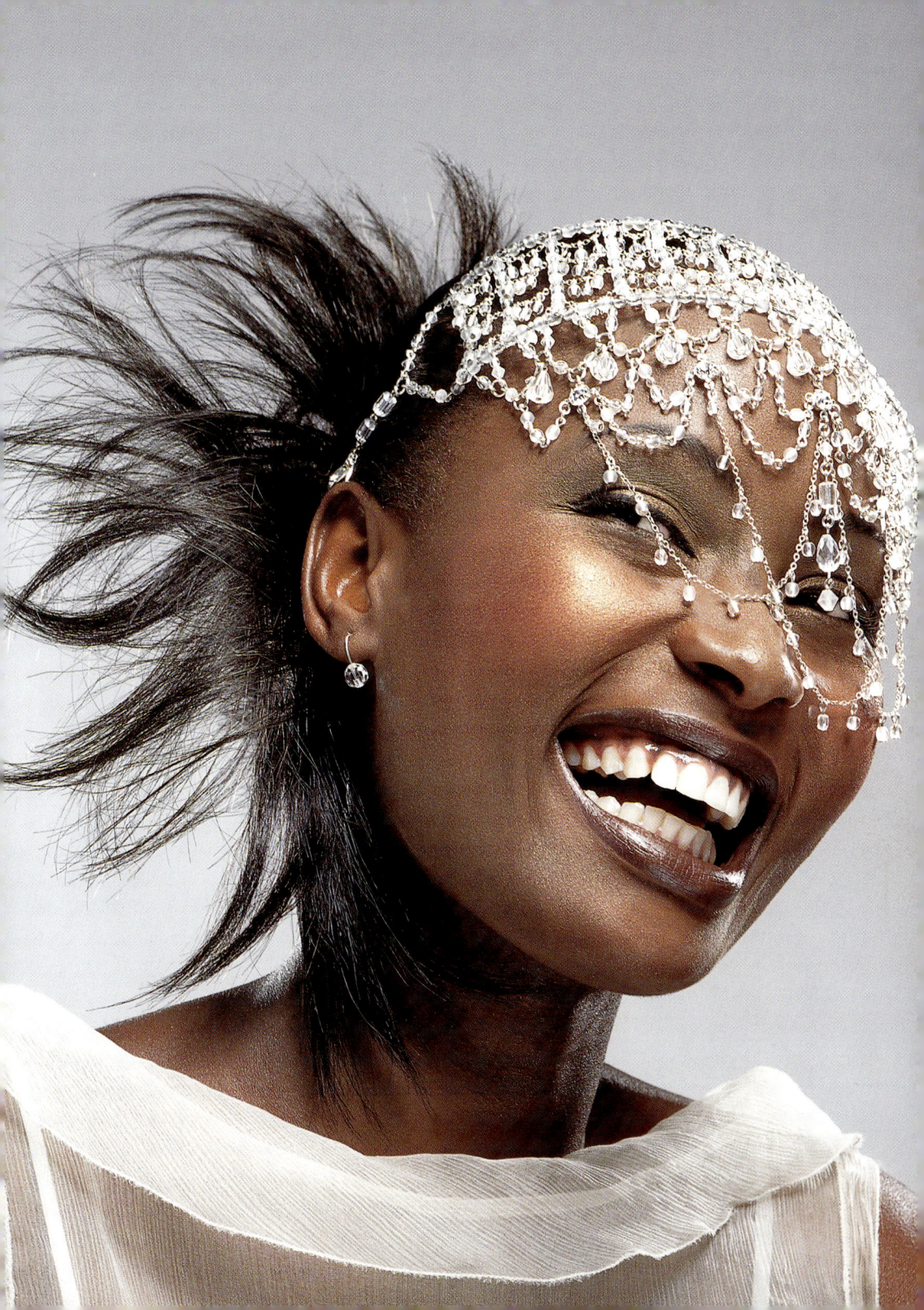

**It's Saturday night** and the girls are rushing around, brushes in hand, music blaring and empty wine bottles starting to gather on the kitchen table.
'Oh god, I look like a sheepdog,' moans Laura, trying to tease her hair, which has reached the highly unpopular 'difficult' stage, into some kind of style. Jaz pops her hair around the bathroom door.

'Want some help?' she offers, looking as if she's never had a bad-hair day in her life. She loves her new style so much that she's left it hanging loose, dressing it up with only a slick of blue hair mascara to enhance the natural glossy blackness. Luckily, her dressing table is still littered with every beauty fix and whimsy on the market. She grabs some hair grips with subtle flowers fashioned from jade and ruby beads. Laura looks dubious as Jaz runs a little texturizing wax through her hair, pulling the shorter sections from the front and twisting them into ridges. Despite Laura's general aversion to all things feminine, she has to admit that Jaz has made a virtue of her hair's unruliness.

## ... the girls get ready to party

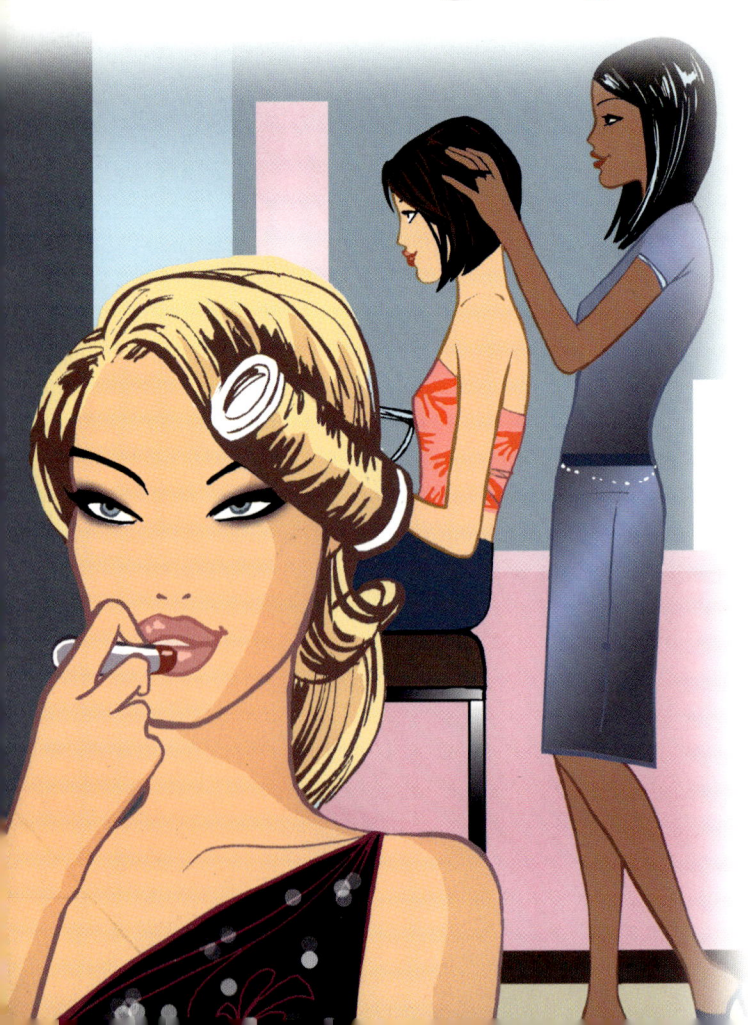

Chrissie limps past with one foot in a tiger-print mule, and spies the missing one poking out from underneath Jaz's bed. Remembering Laura's warning, she bites back her annoyance, only to catch a glimpse of Laura looking fabulous in casual jeans with her hair in a pretty half-updo. Determined not to be outdone by the house tomboy, she stomps back into her room to turn her plaits into something a bit more glamorous.

Chrissie flicks through *Gloss* magazine until she finds a picture of her favourite glam 'do' of the moment – the 1970s-inspired flick. She applies some volumizing mousse to the front section of her long hair, and then winds it around a huge Velcro roller. After a blast of hot air from her hairdryer and a spritz of hairspray, she leaves it to set and gets to work with the lip gloss.

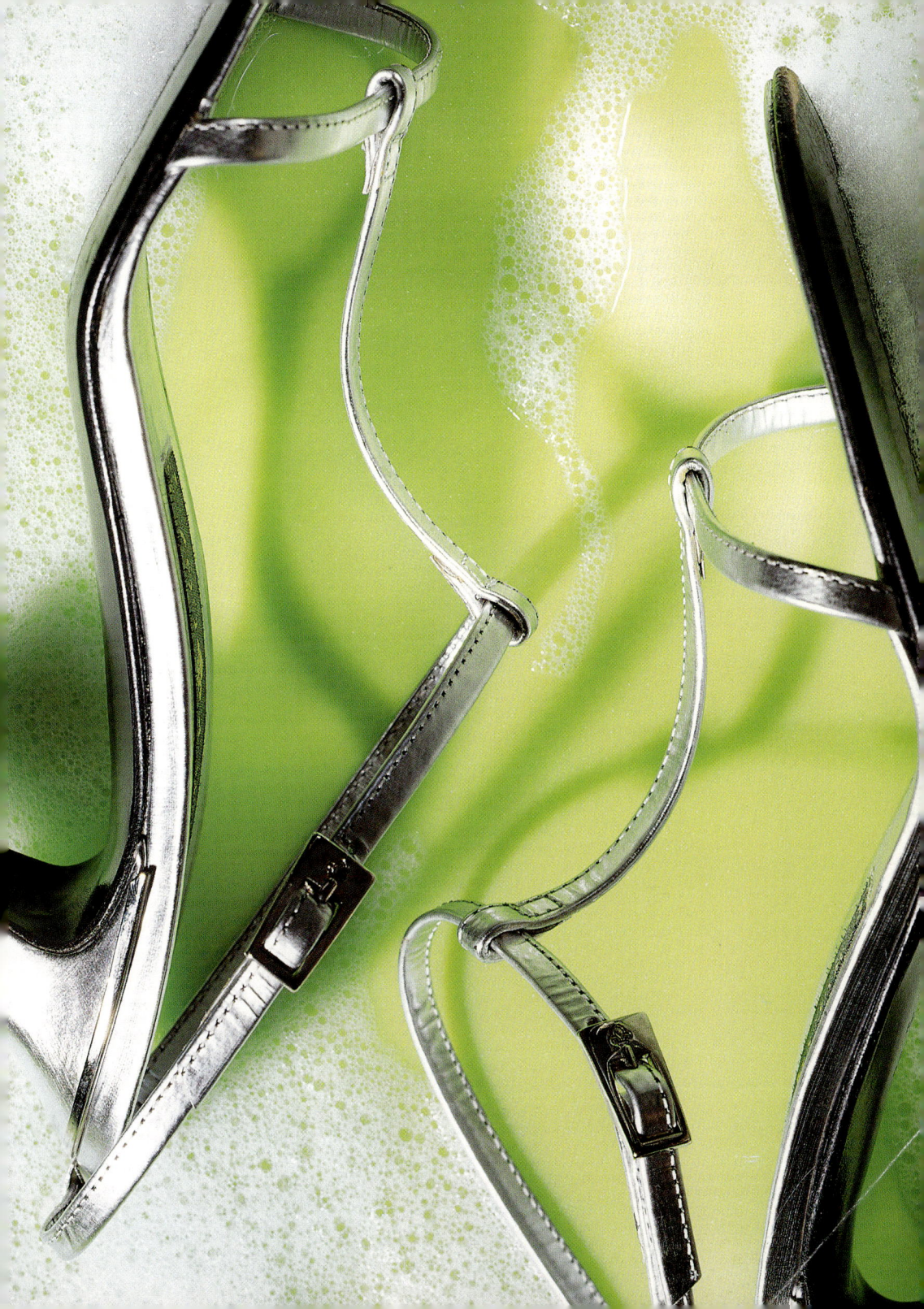

# romantic

This girl is a true romantic. She loves nothing better than watching reruns of *Gone with the Wind* on rainy days – and it never fails to bring tears to her eyes. She's been planning her wedding day for as long as she can remember. Her dress will be fit for a princess – a beautiful full-skirted, tight-bodiced affair with the longest train she can find – and there will be flowers everywhere, in blushing pink and cream.

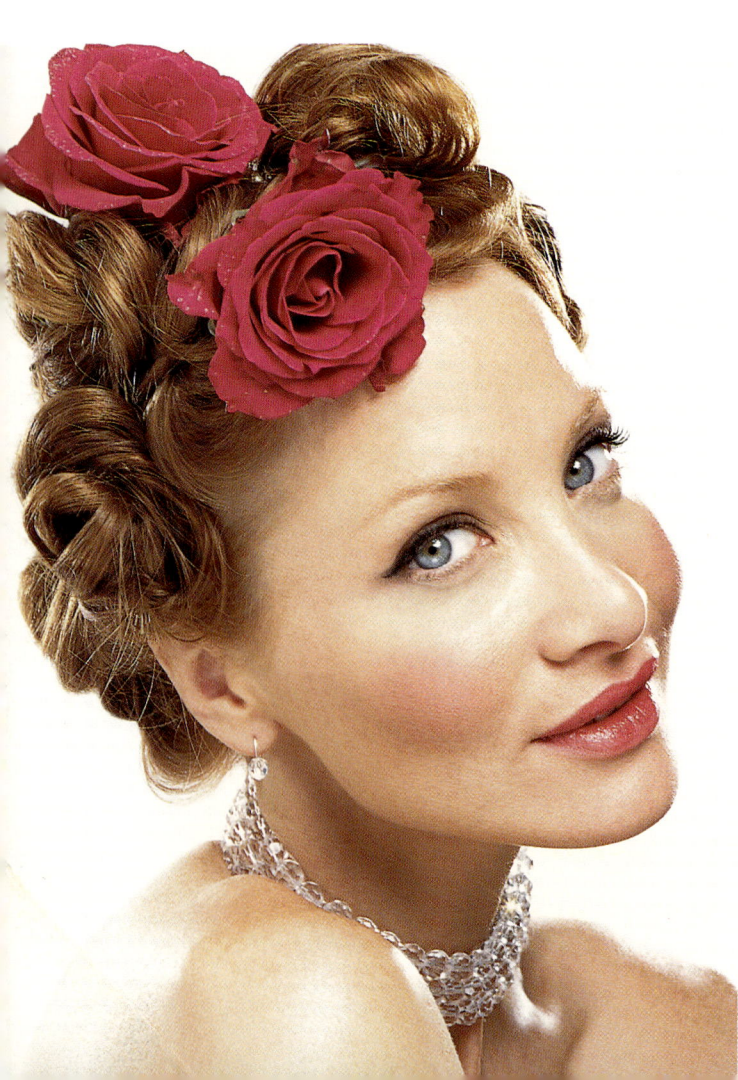

## hair solutions

Long hair will be worn loose and full with a gentle wave and fresh flowers woven into it at the crown. With mid-length hair, fresh tea roses in muted purples and pinks can be used to form a natural Alice band over the crown. You can create a dramatic short-hair look by smoothing hair away from the face with a beaded tiara.

**LEFT AND RIGHT**

This is a very modern take on the classic pin curl. Sections of hair, approximately 5 cm (2 inches) square, are twisted around the fingers and pinned in place all over the head using matt hair grips. Large, fresh flowers are interspersed between the curls.

**OVERLEAF**

Very straight, long hair is tonged using large-barrelled hot tongs to create gentle waves that are left loose to cascade down the back. For added interest a natural flower garland is pinned in place in the centre of the crown.

**HAIR SNIP**

IF YOU ARE USING FRESH FLOWERS IN YOUR HAIR, CAREFULLY SPRITZ THEM WITH WATER USING A VERY FINE SPRAY TO PREVENT THEM FROM DROOPING AND KEEP THEM FRESH ALL DAY LONG.

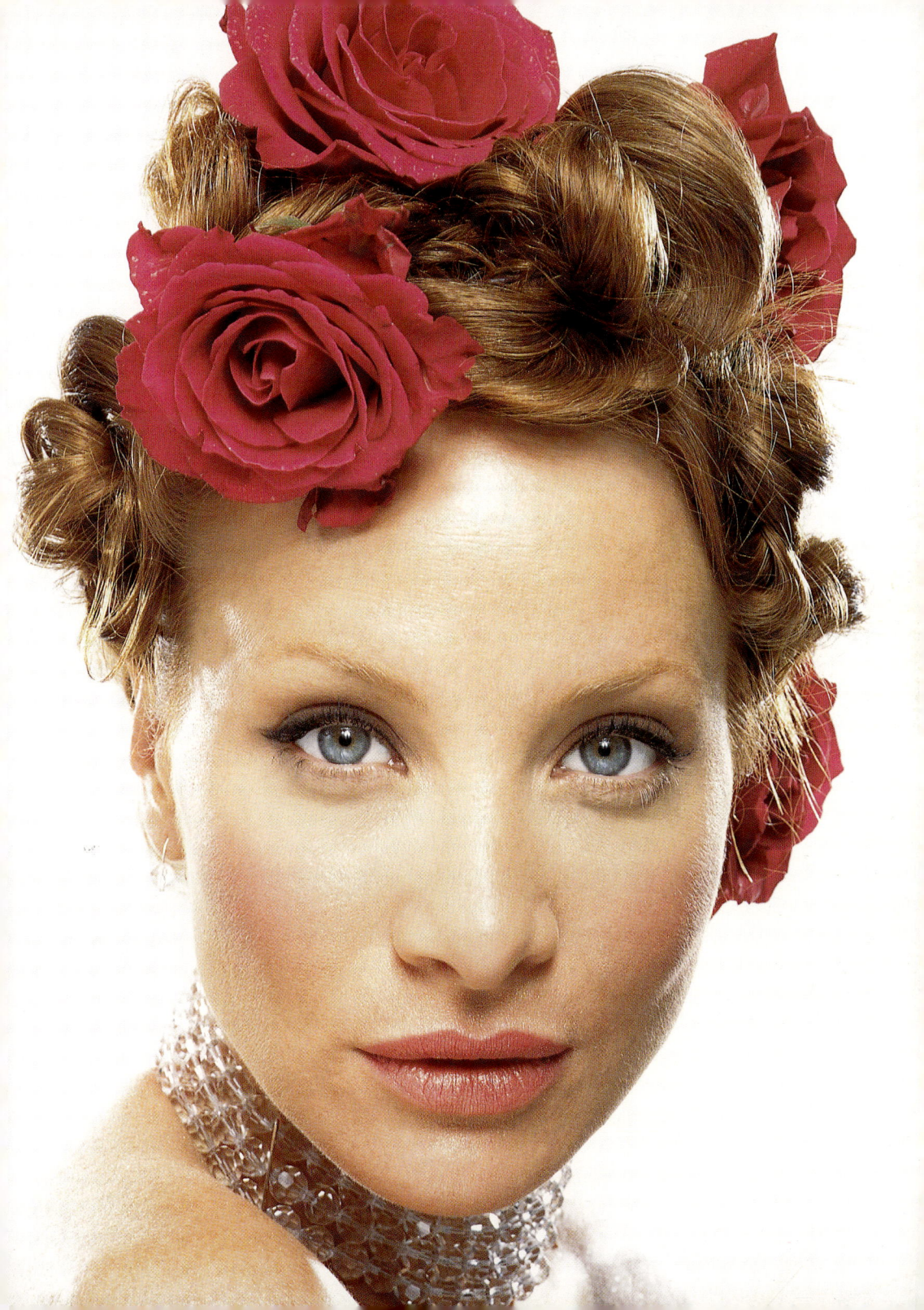

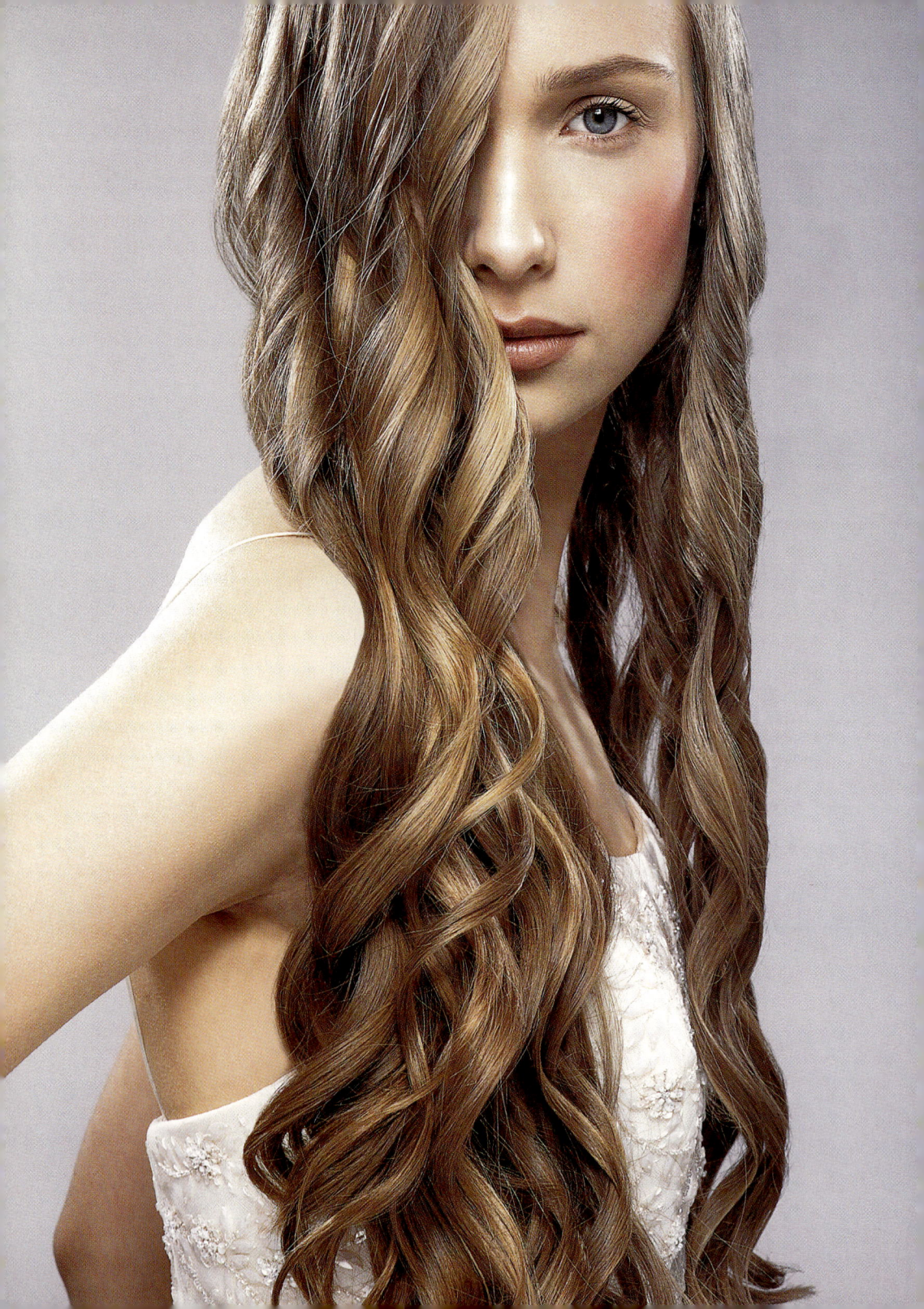

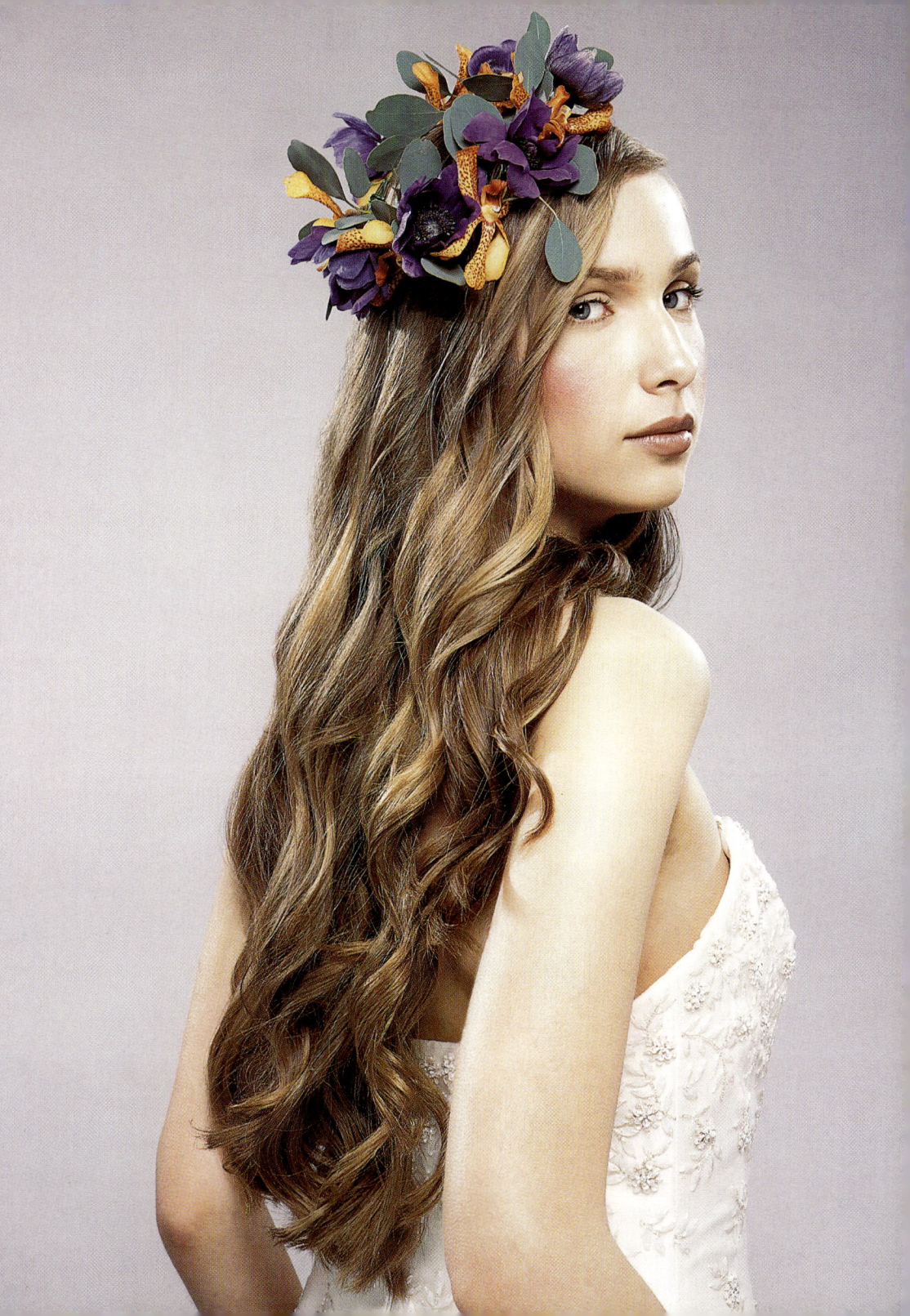

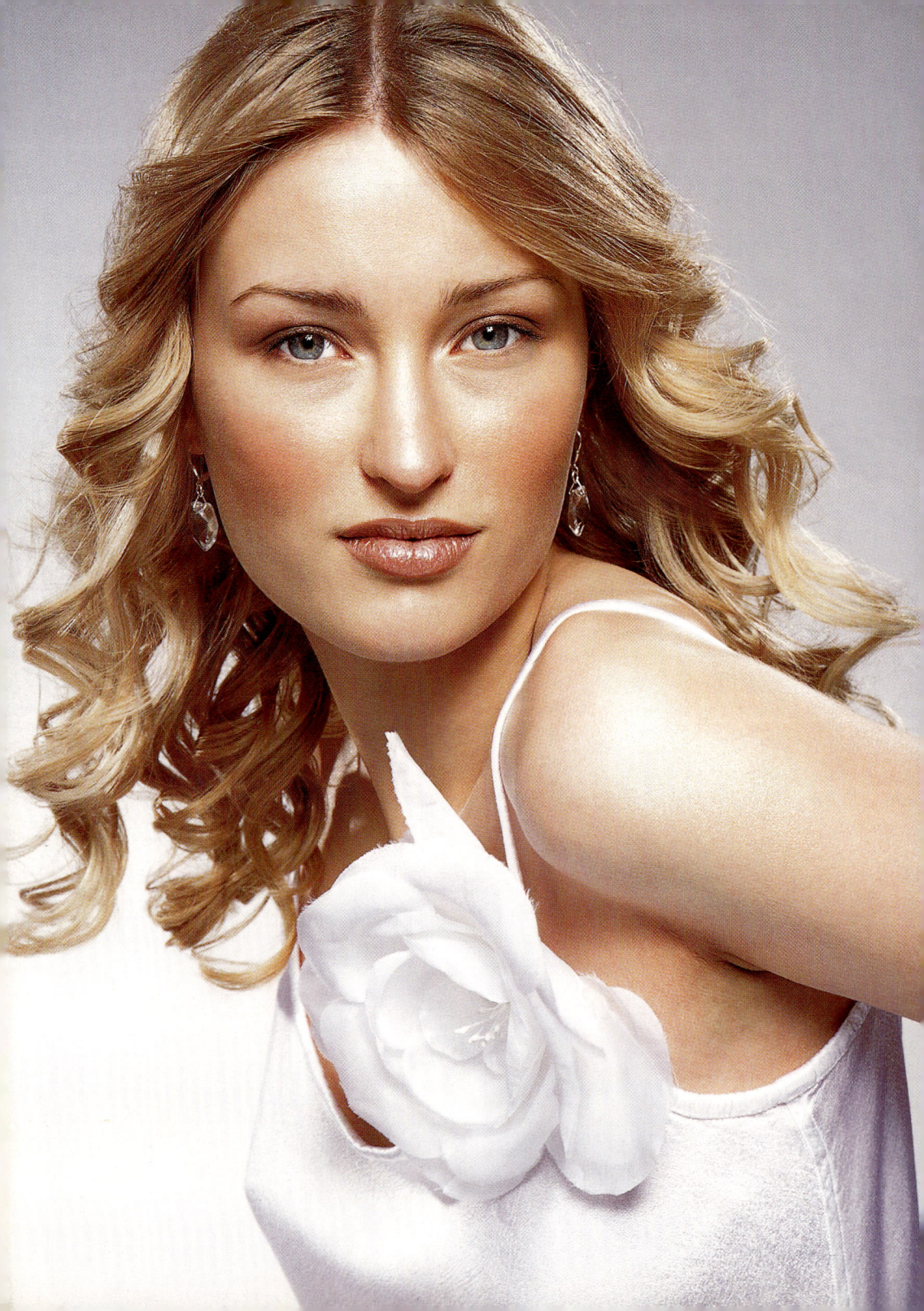

# beach

This fun- and sun-loving girl is the ultimate beach babe, so it's no surprise that she wants a wedding by the sea. She'll wear a strappy white dress or a string bikini and toe rings, with only her parasol to shield her from the rays.

## hair solutions

Minimum fuss with maximum effect is the order of the day here. Whatever your hair length, running some hair oil through your locks will keep it protected from the sun and sea air. Long hair looks great secured in a low bun off to one side at the nape of the neck. Pull some loose ends out to keep it playful. Veils and tiaras are pretty much out, but a big, exotic single bloom can look great tucked behind your ear.

**LEFT AND BELOW LEFT**

The hair is tonged using multi-sized barrelled tongs to give loose romantic ringlets. An anti-humidity blow-dry spray is used to maximize the longevity of the style and also to minimize frizz. Alternatively, the curls can be broken up with a light serum and a comb pulled through the top section and secured above the crown (below left).

**BELOW**

The hair is sectioned into 2.5-cm (1-inch) squares. Ribbons, chosen to match the outfit, are tied around the base of each section of hair and then wrapped around its length in a crisscross formation, keeping the tension all the way down, and tied securely at the ends of the hair. The ends of the ribbons can either be left to hang free, or snipped off for a tidier look.

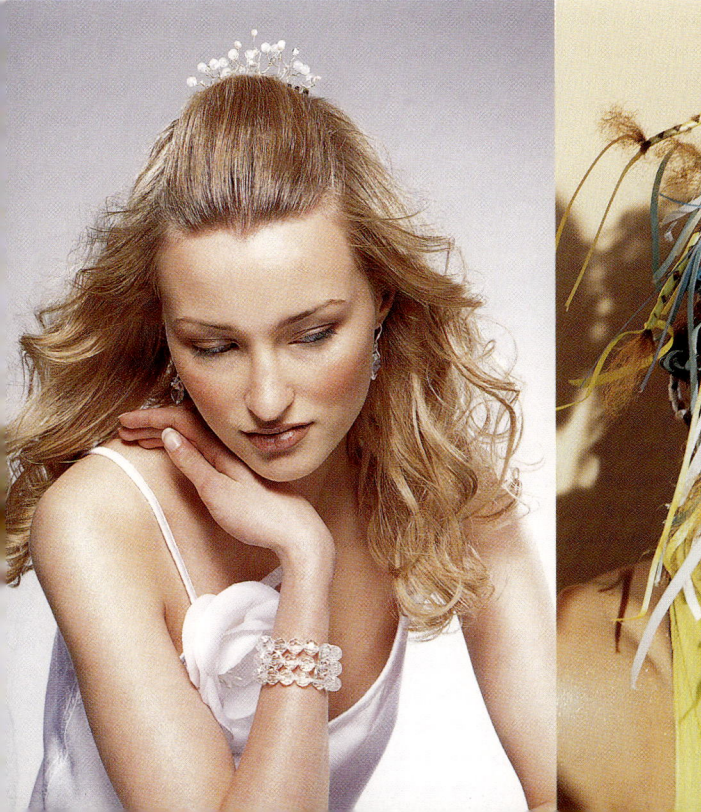

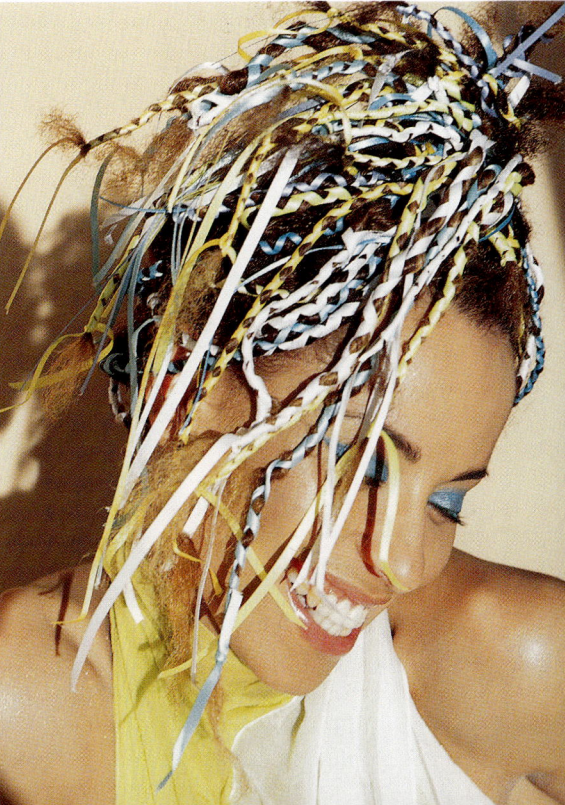

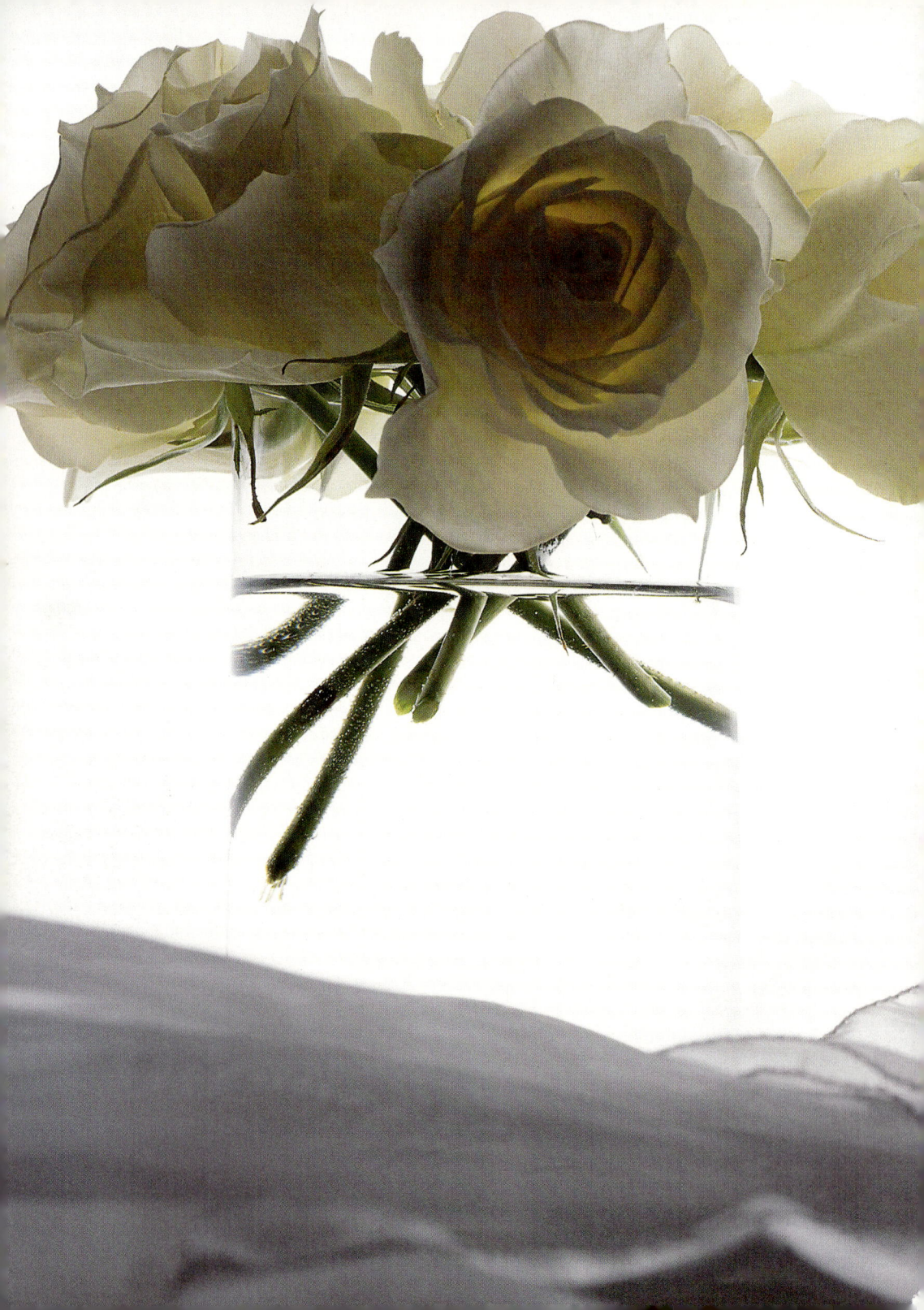

# the big day

# the big day dawns at last ...

'**You are so sly!**' **giggled Polly,** as she accepted a glass of Champagne from Kate. Kate had finally let everyone in on her news – which explained her recent secrecy and absences from the house.

'Well, I wanted to make sure that I'd been accepted before I told you,' she said. 'And also, the course I want to do, the only one that combines nutrition and physiotherapy, is based in Edinburgh ... which means I'll be moving out.' Polly looked up from under the slab of backcombed fringe (bangs) that currently flopped in front of her face.

'I'm glad you've brought that up,' she began, 'because there's something I have to tell you all, too. We've decided to live in London. It'll take at least three months to organize Simon's transfer, so there's plenty of time to make other arrangements.' She looked imploringly at each of her friends.

'Oh, stop looking like Bambi,' said Chrissie. 'We're all big girls, you know, we'll be fine!' Laura nodded in agreement, but secretly wasn't so sure. Things between her and John had been strained recently, and she was concerned that maybe he was starting to go off her. Instead of chatting and laughing away as usual, he seemed withdrawn and anxious.

'Polly, unless you to want to wear your crown around your neck it might be a good idea to keep your head still,' chided Charles affectionately. He had come to Polly's home as a special treat for her big day. Keeping her silky, fine blonde hair in a chignon was going to take all his skill and a few industry tricks. He began by applying thickening spray to the hair and winding it onto large rollers to give as much height and body as possible. After drying the hair, he gave it a burst of hot then cold air to help hold the shape, and then removed the rollers. Charles then scooped back the hair into a classic twist and attached the tiara, a delicate pearl affair, towards the front of the crown. After a fine spray of firm-hold hairspray, Charles stepped back to admire his work. It was the perfect look for Polly, elegant and simple but with enough grandeur to carry off her glamorous gown.

Despite her original concerns about allowing the girls to choose their own dresses and hairstyles, they all looked fantastic. Jaz had chosen a pink dress, tied on one shoulder with an asymmetrical hem. Her sleek black hair followed her hemline, parted to one side and secured with a cluster of pink roses attached to a sequinned clip. She also wore a wrist band of roses. Polly had never seen Laura looking as feminine as she did in her long lilac shift dress with a low, draped back, her hair in a short bob with a band of pale pink roses against her dark hair. Kate had left her hair loose, with roses dotted through its tumbling curls. Her milky complexion was set off perfectly against the pink of her knee-length dress, which, as Jaz had advised had a slightly draped neck. Chrissie, whose natural instinct was to grab attention wherever she could, had chosen a flowing style in pink, with contrasting lilac ruffles and a split starting at mid-thigh. A large rose was pinned behind one ear, pulling back her full blonde hair. The dress had caused Laura to scowl when Chrissie had pulled it off the hanger, but Polly loved it. It was exactly what she would have expected, and it was their differences that she loved them for.

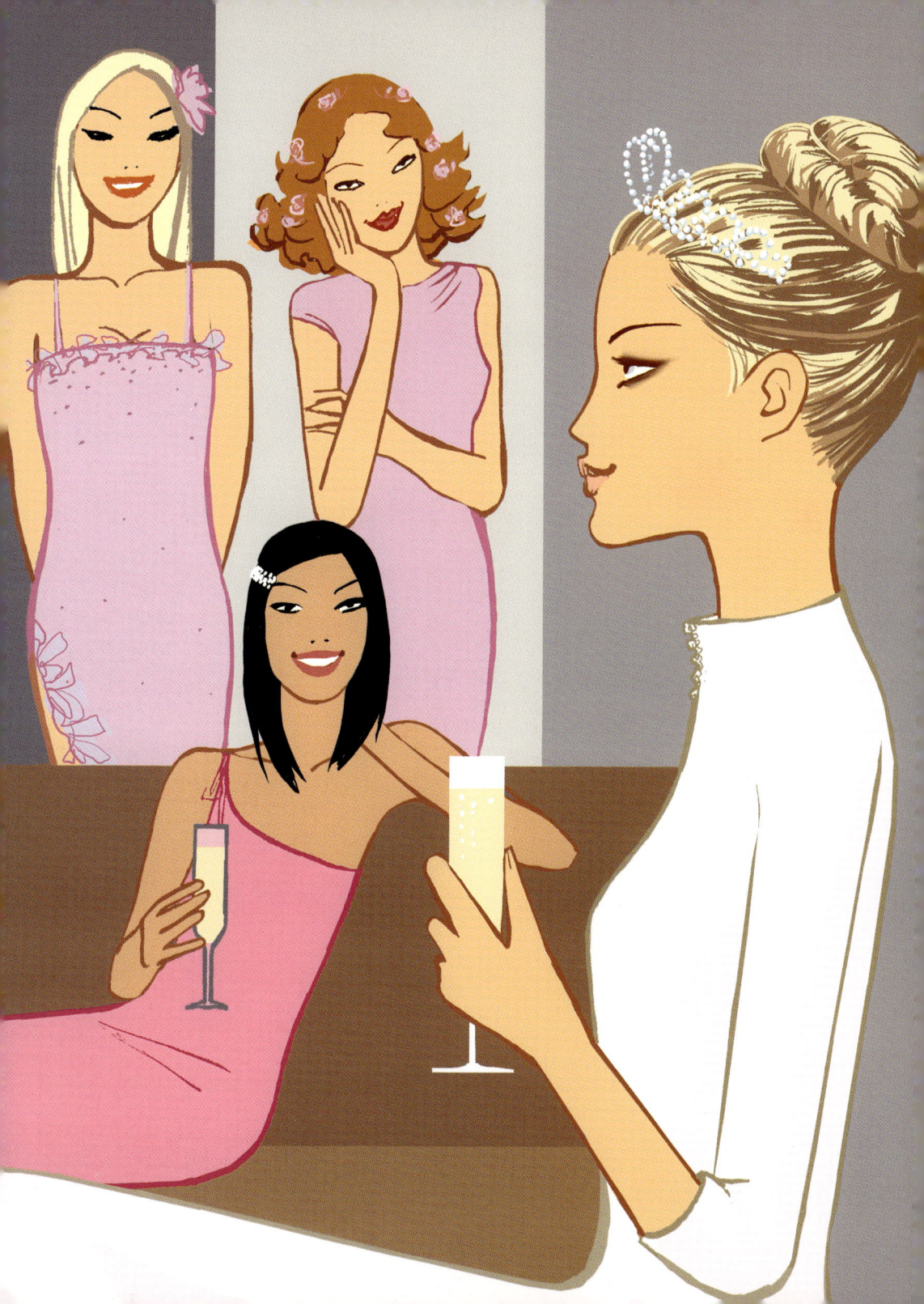

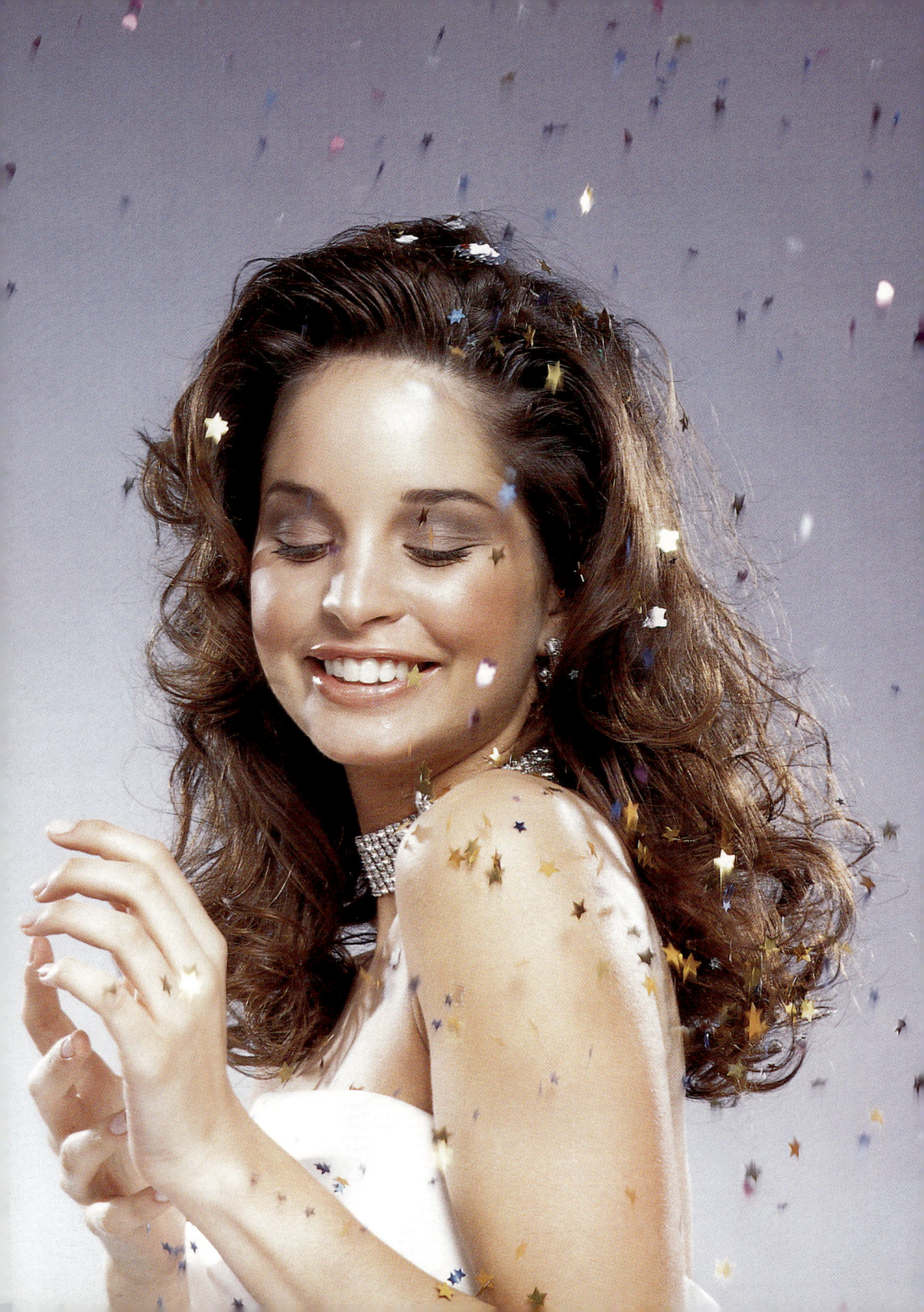

# on the day

Due to all your hard work and preparation, your hair should now be in fabulous condition, ready and waiting to be transformed into your chosen style. Resist the urge to slather on conditioner for a last-minute boost, or fill your hair with extra product – it will only weigh it down. Stick to your tried-and-tested routine.

## entourage

In the same way that you wouldn't leave your bridesmaids' dresses until the last minute, you should also consider in advance how their hairstyles will work with yours. Are you theming your looks and want them to have scaled-down versions of your style? Is this practical? Will they feel more comfortable in a style similar to their normal look?

A key thing to consider is the ages of your bridesmaids. Little girls are usually happy to take instruction, but adult bridesmaids will often have strong feelings about their look. It is sometimes better (and more harmonious) if bridesmaids are allowed to wear their hair – and dresses – in a more individual way (it is also highly unlikely that grown-up bridesmaids will have similar hairstyles). A great way to do this is by using flowers, small tiaras or hair accessories and allowing them to be interpreted in individual ways. Try to create an atmosphere that will allow your bridesmaids to tell you if they are uncomfortable. Ask them to keep a scrapbook of looks they like and see if you can find a compromise.

## products

Although there is a whole array of hair products available to help you achieve your perfect look, they will be most effective if you use fewer of them in the right combination. Remember, the products you use every day may not be right for achieving a more elaborate hairstyle, so make sure you select the right ones.

### mousse
This airy foam will thicken flyaway hair and give control with a natural appearance.

### curl activator
Curly hair can sometimes suffer from lack of moisture, which this product is packed full of. Use it sparingly, though, as too much can turn definition into wet-look.

### gel
Ideal for controlling and volumizing short or fine hair, gel is a bride's best friend. Even if you've never used it before, consider using it for updos and to tame unruly wisps.

### hairspray
The classic mistake for those needing staying power is to spray too much of this stylist's staple, rather than selecting the right holding strength. This will give your hair a hard look and dull its shine. Get the strength right in the first place and it will last.

### styling crème
Some leave-in conditioners also double as a styling crème, which can create a smooth, flat finish. It can also be used on dry ends. Use it sparingly.

### serum
This can be used to control frizz or enhance shine. It is a great way to make the hair look healthily polished, but don't use too much, as it can make the hair look greasy.

### wax and pomade
These range from a hard, shoe polish-like wax to a softer, creamy texture. Use these products to create excellent definition on short hair, and to separate strands and enhance the layers of long hair or a fringe (bangs).

### shine spray
Similar to serum, this can be used on top of other products to restore gloss.

**Ceremony over,** guests greeted and speeches read, Polly slips away to spice up her look for the evening reception, taking the girls for company.

'I hope Simon's parents will recognize you when you return,' giggles Laura, as Jaz produces powders and potions from her seemingly bottomless bag.
'Not that it matters,' says Kate. 'Now that you're Mrs Simon they can hardly call off the wedding.' Polly smiles serenely. Everything had been perfect. It had been a wonderful Indian-summer day; all of the people she loves had been around her, and watching Simon waiting for her at the top of the aisle had given her the best feeling she'd ever known.
'Can you turn into the light a bit Pol?' asks Jaz, removing Polly's tiara and unpinning her chignon as Charles had shown her. She takes a large bristle brush and brushes out the hairspray, letting the hair bounce back in big, soft curls. Grabbing some styling spray from the SOS kit, she sprays Polly's upturned head to help maintain body. Jaz smoothes back the top front section, and holds it in place with a crystal beaded slide, creating a 1950s-inspired half-up, half-down style.

# ... polly's day-to-night transformation

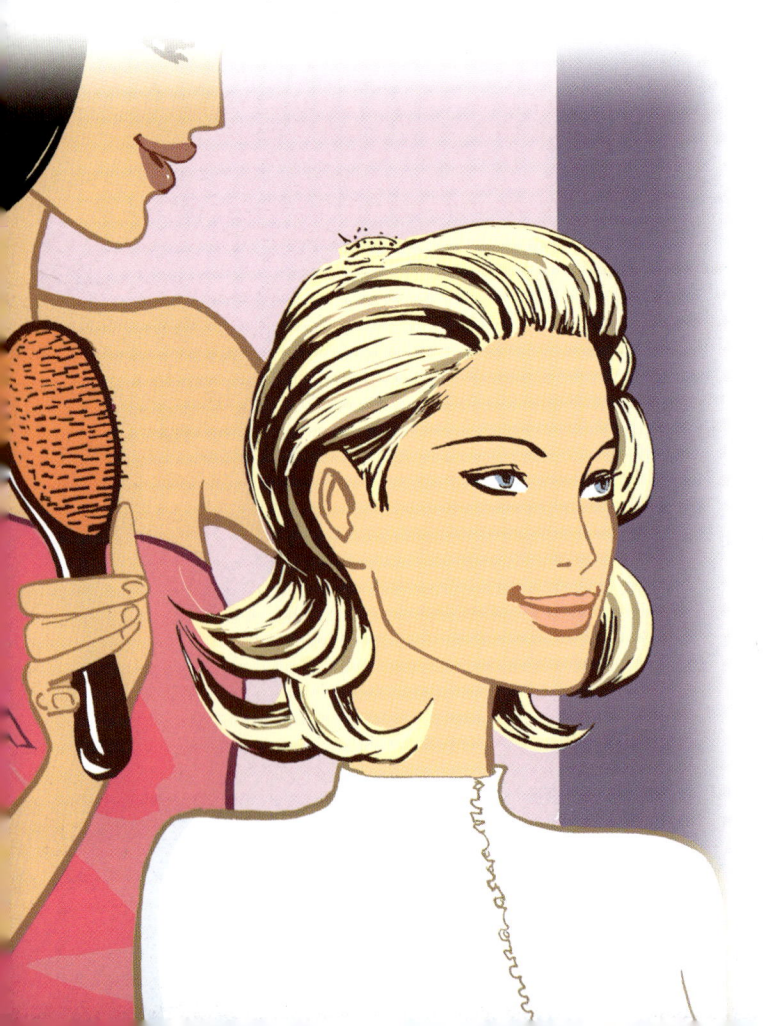

'Don't go too crazy with the gold look,' Polly warns Jaz, who had promised to create a spectacular night-time look for her. In moments of pre-wedding anxiety she had imagined leading the first dance with glittery striped cheekbones. 'You lot have such little faith in me,' says Jaz, slipping a glitter stick back into her make-up bag. 'When have I ever been Over The Top?' The girls cackle wildly as they remind each other of Jaz's more extreme forays into fashion – her tie-dyed hair, her luminous fishnet tights ... Jaz just smiles and begins dusting shimmering gold powder on Polly's cheekbones and hair. After an extra layer of mascara and a touch of eyeliner to enhance Polly's blue eyes, she slicks some clear gloss across her lips, a look that's glamorous without being heavy. 'OK, you comedians,' she says, standing back to admire her handy work. 'It's time to get Mrs Simon back to her party.'

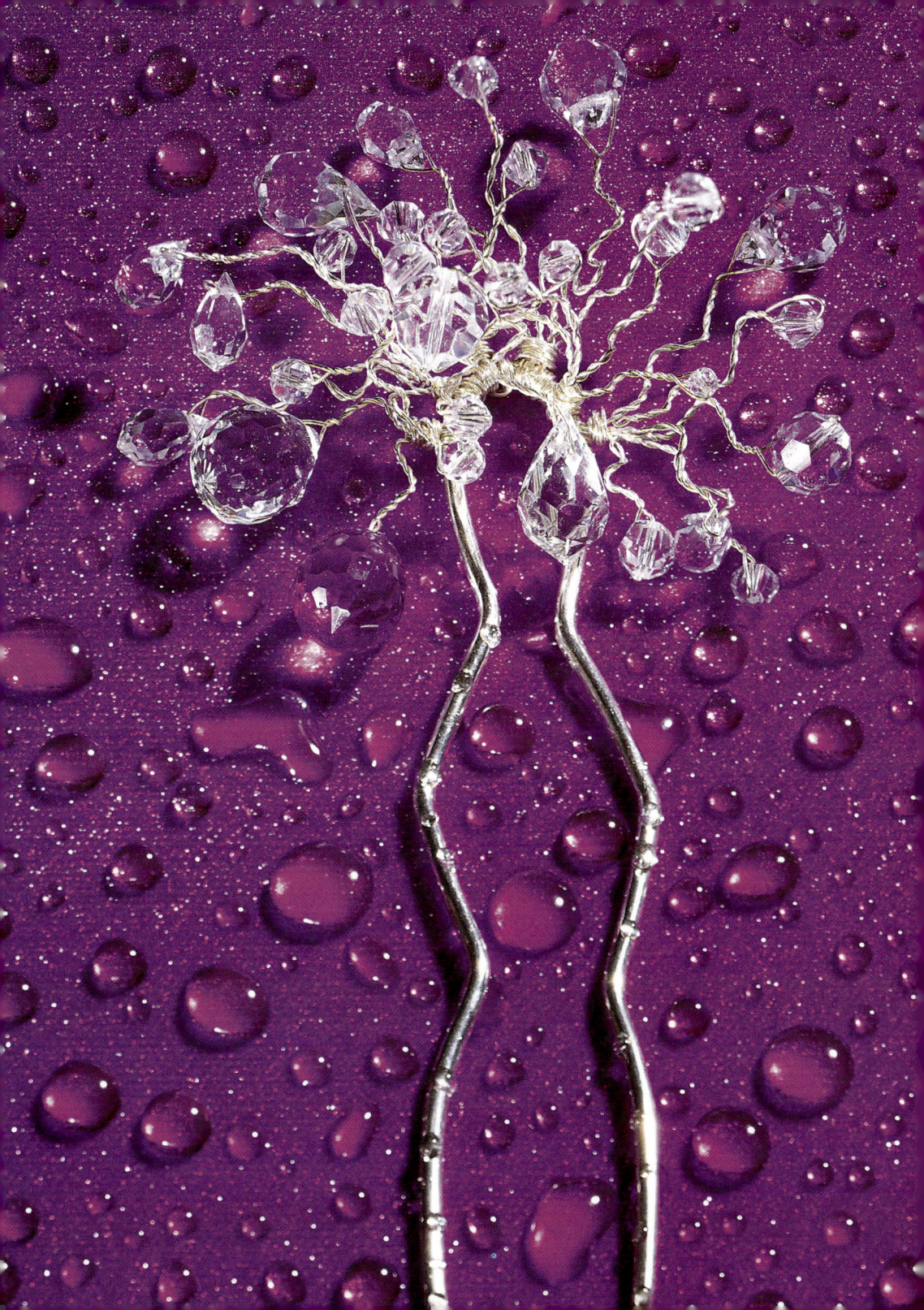

# making it last

Whether you are doing your own wedding hair or visiting your stylist, there are certain tricks that will give your hair extra staying power. Make sure your bridesmaids and mother read these tips, too!

**1** If you are having an updo, wash your hair the night before the wedding, rather than on the day, since just-washed hair can be harder to tame. Those with a fringe (bangs) may want to part the front section and wash that separately.

**2** When you use any styling product, it is very important that most of it is applied at the roots, not the ends. This will stop the hair from being too flat.

**3** Silky hair that usually hangs loose in a pretty but stubborn curtain can be tamed by the addition of styling agents. Thickening volumizing spray, wax and mousse will all help the tiara or veil grip onto the hair. Make sure that you do not overcondition fine hair, as this will weigh it down.

**4** To put more volume into your style, alternate between hot and cold heat settings when you are blow-drying your hair. Dry the hair first using hot air, then give each section a cold blast – this will set in body and bounce as the hair cools down and will help to hold the style in shape for longer.

**5** Extra-large rollers will create great volume. Work from the top to the bottom of the head, taking sections of hair that are approximately 2.5–5 cm (1–2 inches) wide, depending on its length and health. Roll the hair under in the direction you want the style to lay and ensure that the rollers sit snugly against the scalp for maximum body. Once all the rollers have been inserted, spritz the hair with a styling spray for long-lasting root lift.

**6** Roller-set your hair to make it more manageable and easier to put up on the day.

**7** When using hair products, try to choose them all from the same range for the most effective results – they are designed to work together.

**8** Backcombing is the backbone of all updos, giving both volume and staying power. It may look bad for your hair but it is essential.

Having a trial run with your veil and tiara is extremely important. Clear combs are the most effective way of securing a veil discreetly and firmly, and you may need to employ matt grips in a shade similar to your hair colour for extra support. Tiaras often come with hooks for slides to be slipped into or with a comb to grip the hair as part of their design. Give your style a serious workout to make sure it has staying power; you will be miserable if you find yourself anxiously trying to balance a slipping tiara all day. Backcombing often helps give the hair texture to which things can grip, as will using product in the hair. Always ask the store from which you buy your veil or tiara to show you how to secure it – they are the experts.

## SOS kit

No bride should venture into the elements without her SOS kit. Take whatever you need to feel secure, then nominate your bridesmaid with the biggest handbag to look after it.

Hairspray and shine spray
Matt hair grips and hair pins – and plenty of them
Natural-bristle smoothing brush
Tail comb
Hot rollers
Bun ring
Hairpiece

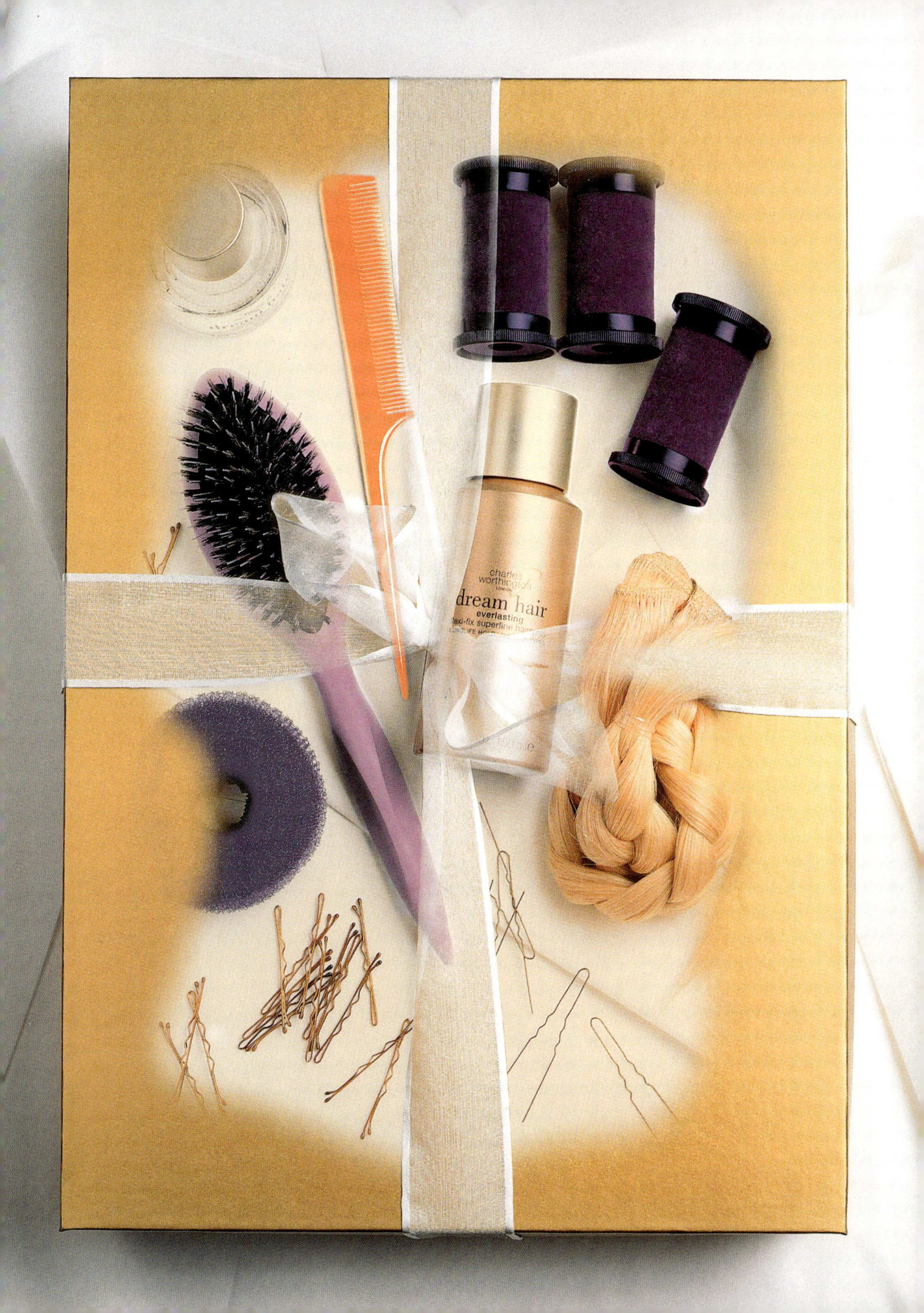
charles worthington
dream hair
everlasting

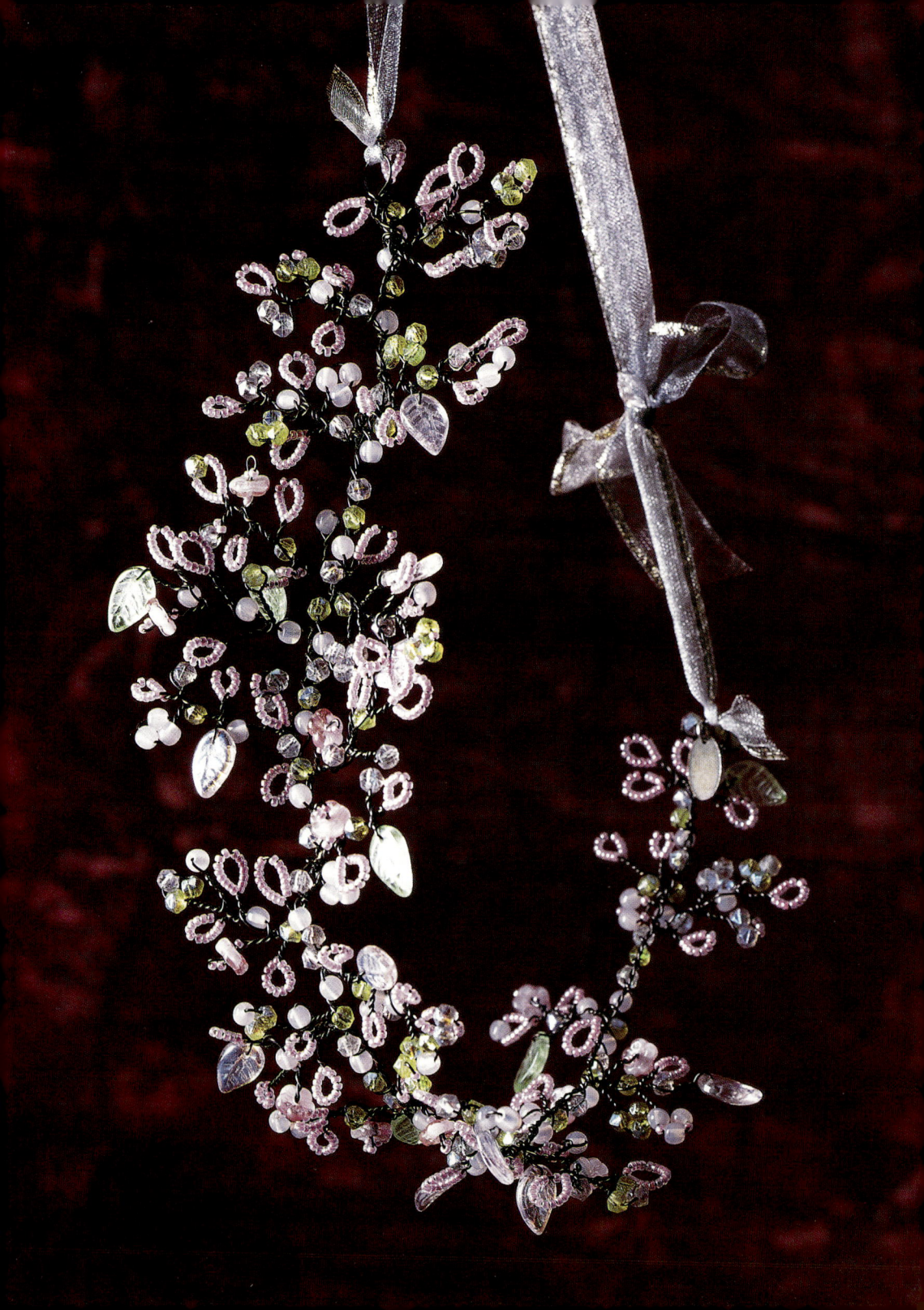

'**I can't believe** I'm doing this,' mutters Chrissie, as she prepares to dash out into the rain to collect Polly's bag from the car. The weather has finally broken, the clear skies turning black with heavy showers. After five minutes in the doorway of the country hotel where the reception is being held, she finally accepts that she'll just have to make a run for it.

The 20-second round trip leaves her completely soaked. Her hair is plastered to her head and her lovely dress is glued to her skin. As she slinks through the door, hugging the wall, and starts up the stairs to the suite, she spots Knell Kendrew, the head of Devastation Records arriving at the reception. She could weep on the spot. Never one to indulge in soul-searching, Chrissie's finally realized what

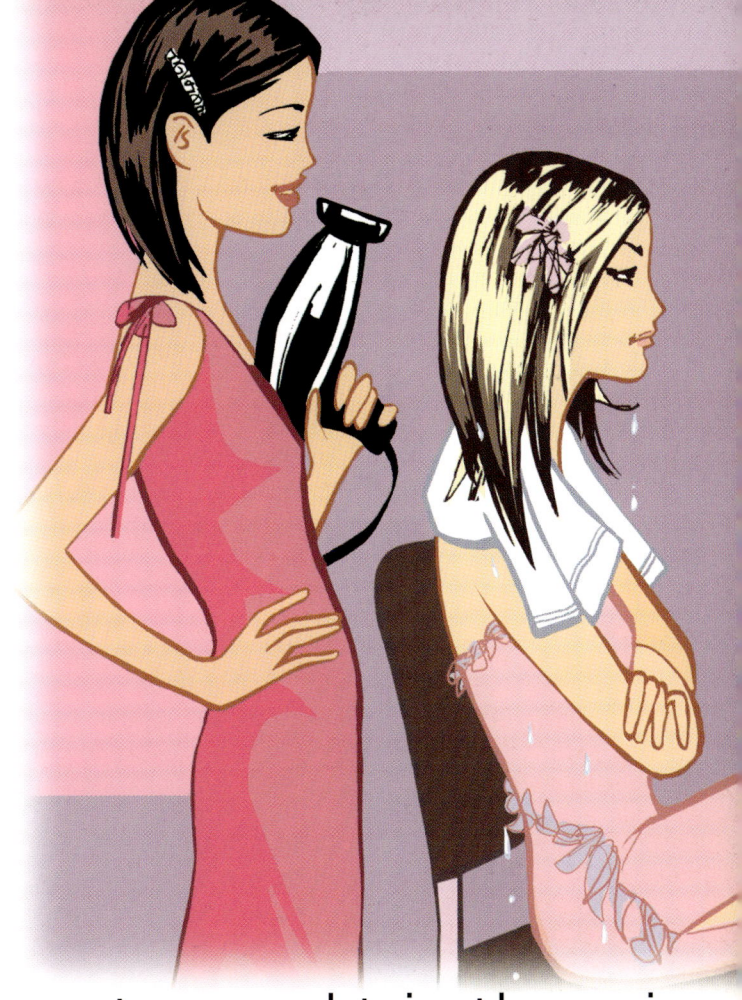

## ... chrissie gets caught in the rain

has been making her so touchy of late. It seems that everyone else is moving on in their lives, while she's left stuck behind the reception desk at Devastation Records, waiting for the big break that never seems to come.

'There you are! You're soaked and it's completely my fault!' cries Polly, making her way down the stairs towards her, in her freshly made-up perfection.

'Don't panic anyone,' says Jaz, rummaging in her bag with one hand and nudging Chrissie into the suite with the other. 'Charles left me an SOS kit for exactly this kind of crisis. Get that dress off.'

Once inside, Chrissie wriggles out of her wet dress, drapes it on the radiator and shrugs on one of the fluffy white dressing gowns hanging on the door. She takes a seat at the dressing table and begins removing her melting mascara. Jaz combs some shine spray from Charles's SOS kit through the length of Chrissie's hair. With some deft twisting, she pulls it back into a band, folds the hair over and secures it into a low, loose bun, with a few strands pulled out. The effect is pretty and sexy – the perfect match for her ruffled dress. Maybe she isn't going to have to hide from Knell after all.

THE BIG DAY 75

// THE BIG DAY

# post-ceremony

Once the ceremony is over, a grand style may seem slightly extreme, so perform a quick transformation by detaching your veil and leaving your tiara in place.

## day to night

For a different evening look, make sure your daytime style can translate easily into night-time glamour. Too much product will leave the hair lank and dull, so use one that will brush out easily, such as hairspray. Take a bridesmaid with you when trying out looks so that she can see how your style needs to be changed, using your own SOS kit.

**LEFT**
The hair is divided into 2.5-cm (1-inch) square sections, and each one is bound with thin copper wire which allows you to sculpt the tendrils into the desired shape. Finish off with a simple accessory.

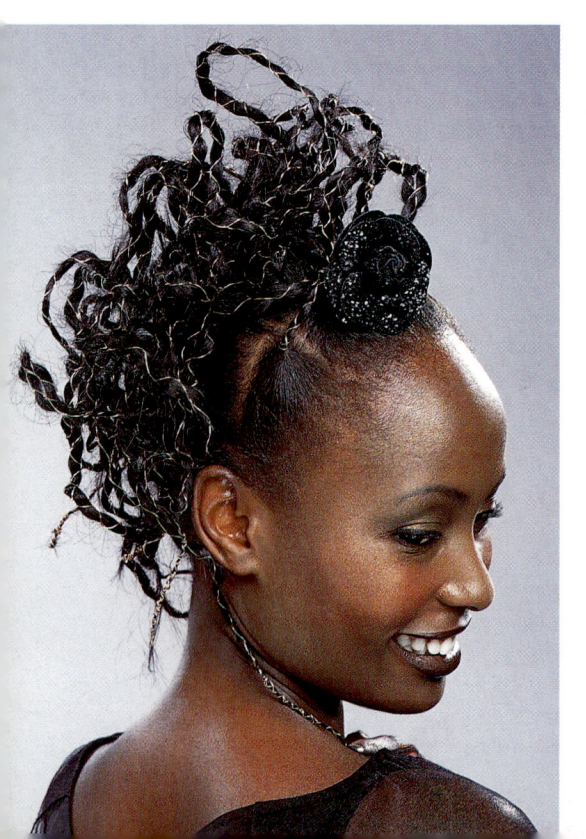

## going away

If you are travelling as soon as the reception is over, you'll want a hairstyle that is tidy and manageable. If you have long hair, try a chic, simple ponytail or scooped-up chignon, while a smudge of wax is great for tousling or slicking back short hair. Some wedding-day hairstyles are likely to leave your hair kinky and unmanageable when you remove all the grips and paraphernalia. Happily, this means that you can employ the classic going-away style – the Grace Kelly headscarf.

**RIGHT**
For this glamorous 'Jackie O' look, the hair is set on large heated rollers to give volume and wave, and then backcombed at the roots to create big-impact hair. Finish off with a spritz of hairspray to hold.

### post-ceremony hair tips

Plan your day-to-night and going-away styles before the day. You may need to buy extra kit.

If your wedding-day hairstyle looks fine with your going-away outfit, don't change it for the sake of it.

Keep it simple – by the time you leave the reception, you won't want to fuss over something complicated.

Don't be tempted to add lots more extra product – it will only make your hair look limp and dull.

Make sure you can travel with your hairstyle – you don't want to have to sit bolt upright on a long flight.

Take your SOS kit with you in your hand luggage.

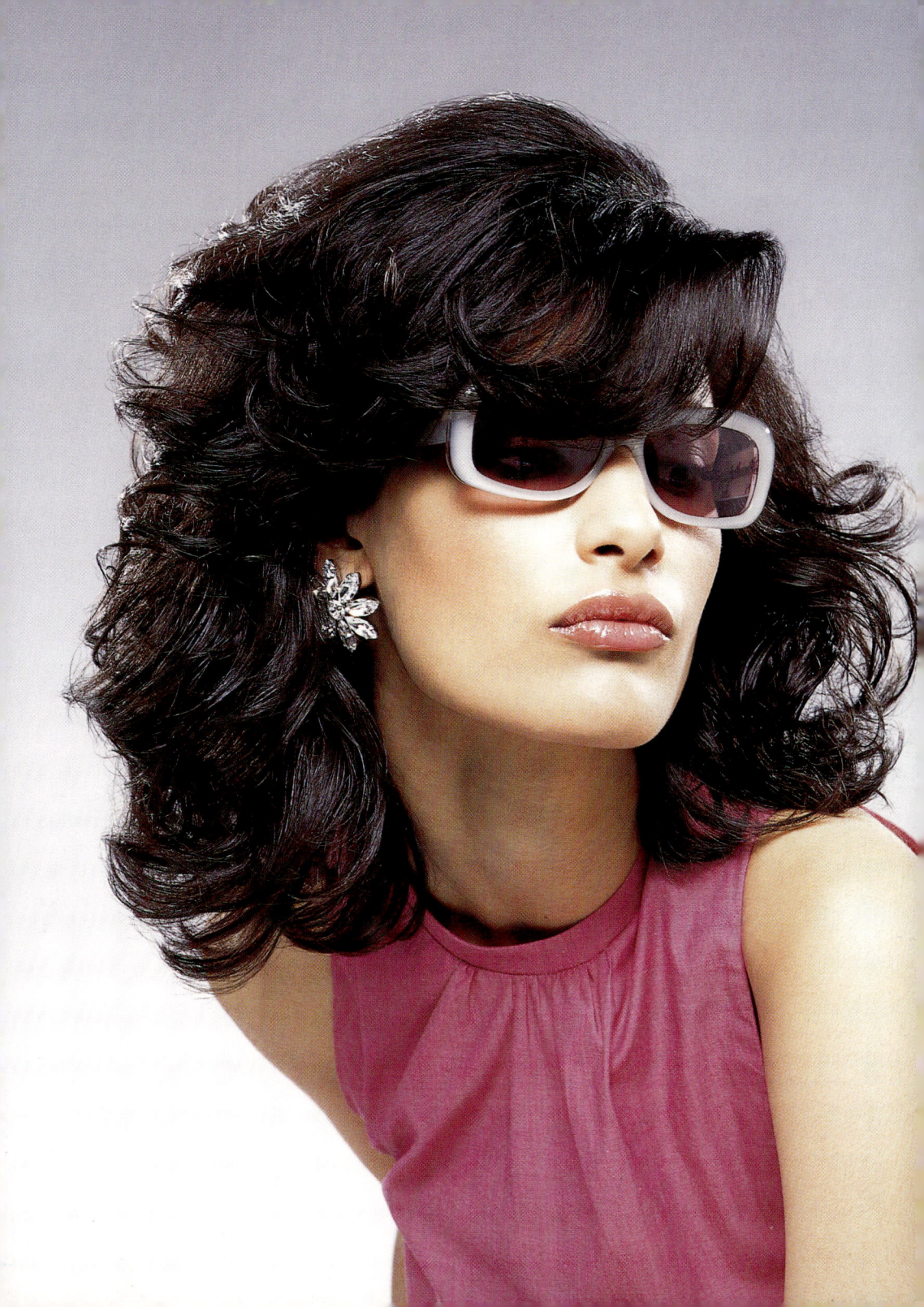

# happily ever after ...

**All of the girls,** except Chrissie, were hovering in the doorway of the plush country hotel, waiting for the happy couple to make their exit.

'Well, I think we should move to East London. That's where everything happens these days; don't you think so, Laura?' said Jaz. Laura mumbled non-commitally. She had hoped that maybe she wouldn't be sharing a house anymore – at least, not with her girlfriends. But judging from John's mood this evening, he seemed less likely to want to co-habit than inhabit another country altogether.

'Oh, look!' cried Kate, breaking her train of thought, 'Here they come!' Kisses, tears, hugs and more confetti rained down on the wedding party as the couple slowly made their way through the crowd. Jaz looked around frantically, 'Where is Chrissie? She's going to miss them!' On cue, Chrissie came bobbing through the crowd. An arm reached out and pulled her out of the throng. It was Knell.

'Chrissie?' she said. Chrissie looked up at Knell, the most powerful woman at Devastation Records, and smiled nervously. She was unsure how to respond to the older woman, knowing that her looks and flirty charms would have no effect.

'Oh, hi Knell, what are you doing here?' she managed to ask.

'Simon's good friends with my son,' Knell explained. 'They were at university together in the States. Anyway, I'm glad to have bumped into you here, I've seen a different side to you this evening.'

'Yeah, I bet you have,' thought Chrissie gloomily. Herself wearing a wrinkled dress and her make-up washed off by a torrential downpour was not the kind of lasting impression she wanted to linger with Knell. 'I suppose you wondered why you didn't get the gig with Pout,' Knell continued, referring to Chrissie's unsuccessful audition for a girl band earlier in the year. 'It was because you didn't bring anything new and different. Basically, you were the same as the girls already in the band – all polish and perfection.' Chrissie winced internally, reminded of why Knell was regarded as one of the toughest women in the industry. Knell placed an arm around her shoulders, 'But seeing you tonight has made me reconsider. Maybe what you need is a change of image ... something more natural. People are growing tired of the same old manufactured girl-band line-up. Come and see me on Monday, we'll talk.' Knell gently pushed Chrissie back into the crowd, signifying that their meeting was over. Chrissie continued her struggle to get to the girls in a state of shock. Maybe she was going to get her shot at the limelight after all, and, even better, she wasn't going to have to share it!

'Quick, here they come,' squealed Kate grabbing handfuls of confetti and throwing them into the air. The girls kissed and hugged the happy couple, tears flowing and giggles erupting – Polly was married, like a proper grown-up!

As the car drove off towards the airport, Chrissie turned back to the other three left behind. 'OK,' she said, 'let's go and get some big glasses of Champagne and toast the loss of another single girl.' They started off inside. 'Oh, not you, Laura,' said Jaz, putting her hand to her mouth apologetically. 'You've got to go and see John, he's waiting for you in the rose garden. I forgot to tell you, sorry.'

'Why?' asked Laura, nervously.

'I'm not sure,' cried Jaz over her shoulder. 'He just said he had something to ask you ...'

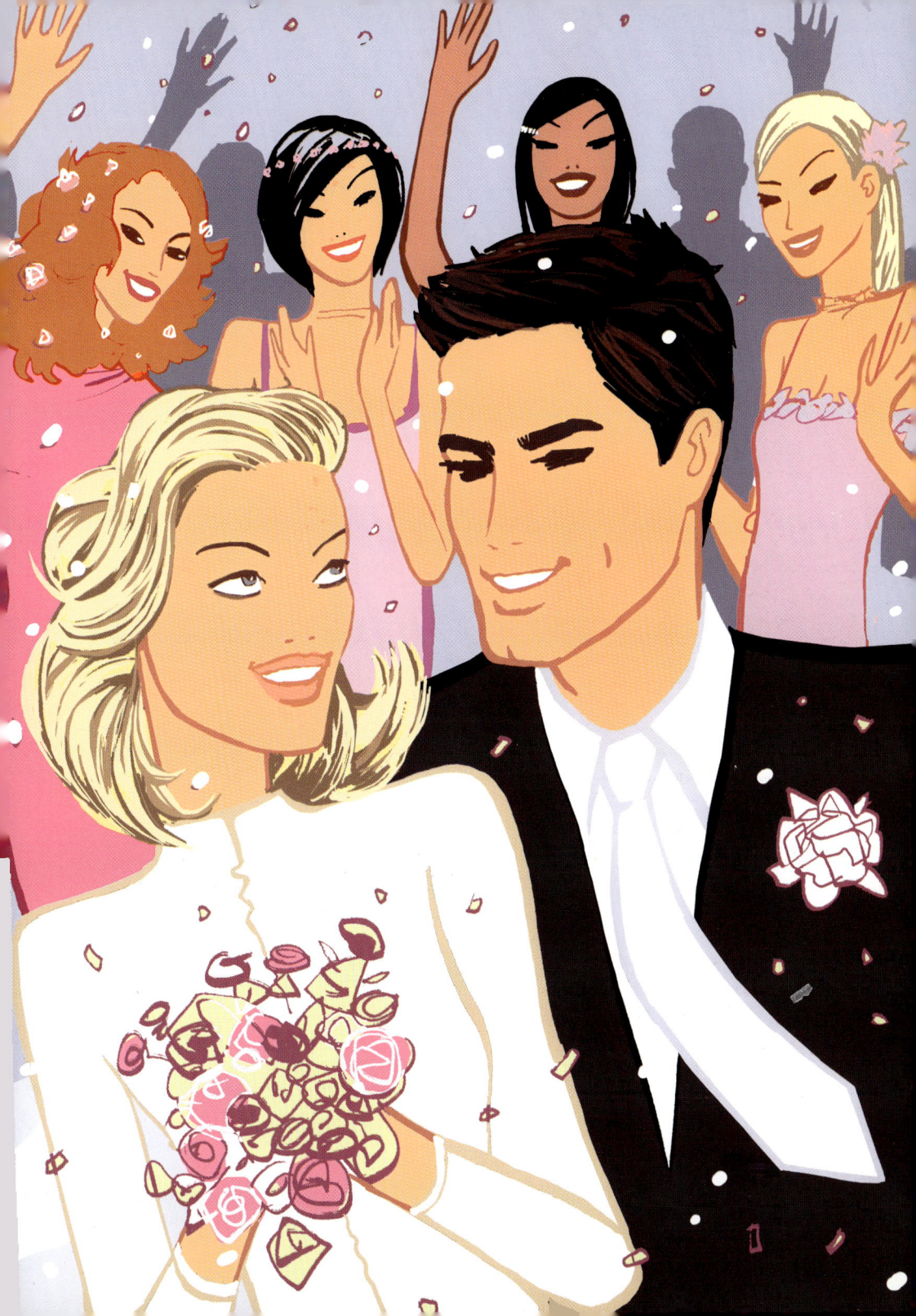

# acknowledgements

Thank you to Adam Reed at the Percy Street salon. With special thanks to Julie Gibson Jarvie, Penny Stock and Venetia Penfold, without whom the book wouldn't have been possible.

With special thanks to the following:

Isabel Kurtenbach Designs (by appointment only), tel: 020 7854 9647, email: design@isabelkurtenbach.com, website: www.isabelkurtenbach.com

Nicola Pulvertaft (by appointment only), tel: 07747 792 082

Amanda Wakeley, 80 Fulham Road, London SW3 6HR, tel: 020 7590 9105

Basia Zarzycka (by appointment only), 52 Sloane Square, London SW1W 8AX, tel: 020 7730 1660, email: basia@basia.com, website: www.basias.com

Butler & Wilson, 20 South Molten Street, London W1K 5QY, tel: 020 7409 2955

Flowers by Bud (by appointment only), tel: 020 8537 0626